ADVANCED STRATEGY FOR MEDICAL PRACTICE L
OPERATIONS MANAGEMENT EDITION

MGMA
104 INVERNESS TERRACE EAST
ENGLEWOOD, CO 80112-5306
877.275.6462
MGMA.COM

Inspiring
healthcare
excellence.℠

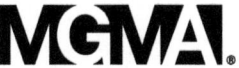

Medical Group Management Association® (MGMA®) publications are intended to provide current and accurate information and are designed to assist readers in becoming more familiar with the subject matter covered. Such publications are distributed with the understanding that MGMA does not render any legal, accounting, or other professional advice that may be construed as specifically applicable to individual situations. Neither representations nor warranties are made concerning the application of legal or other principles discussed by the authors to any specific factual situation, nor is any prediction made concerning how any particular judge, government official, or other person will interpret or apply such principles. Specific factual situations should be discussed with professional advisors.

Editors, Ryan Reaves and Andy Stonehouse

Published by: Medical Group Management Association (MGMA) Library of Congress Control Number: 2022905959

Item: 1049
ISBN: 978-1-56829-043-0

Copyright © 2024 Medical Group Management Association

All rights reserved. No part of this publication may be reproduced, stored in a retrieval system, or transmitted in any form or by any means, electronic, mechanical, photocopying, recording, or otherwise, without the prior written permission of the copyright owner.

Printed in the United States of America

10 9 8 7 6 5 4 3 2 1

Advanced Strategy for Medical Practice Leaders

Volume 1: Financial Management Edition

Volume 2: Human Resources Management Edition

Volume 3: Operations Management Edition

Contents

Contributors xv

Introduction xxi

Chapter 1: Defining the Heart of your Organization 1

    1.1 Introduction 1

    1.2 Mission, Vision and Values 1
        Mission Statement 2
        Vision Statement 2
        Values 3
        MVV Sets the Tone for Your Organization's Success ... 4
        How to Align MVV with Your Organization's Goals ... 4
        The Vital Role of Consistency in Cultivating Culture ... 6

    1.3 Identifying and Engaging Key Players to Achieve Success 7
        Engaging Key Stakeholders During Change 8

    1.4 Operational Excellence and Quality Improvement 10
        Lean and Six Sigma in Healthcare 10
        Process Improvement Tools 12
        Engaging Your Team in Quality Improvement 14
        MIPS and Quality Metrics 15
        Cultivating a Culture of High-Quality Care 15

    1.5 Practice in Action 16

    1.6 Summary 17

Chapter 2: Administrative Structures in Medical Practice Operations 21

2.1 Introduction 21
Importance of Administrative Structures 22

2.2 Leadership's Influence on Administrative Structures 23
Successful Leadership Approach to Administrative Structures 23

2.3 Organizational Design and Structure 24

2.4 Choosing the Right Organizational Structure 27

2.5 Implementing Health Information Systems 28
Identify Needs and Customize Technology 28
Emphasize Adaptability and Continuous Improvement 29

2.6 Financial Management 29
Budgeting and Financial Planning 30
Revenue Cycle Management (RCM) 30
Accounts Receivable Management 31
Strategies for Cost Optimization and Revenue Enhancement 32

2.7 Enhancing Patient Engagement and Satisfaction 33

2.8 Navigating Legal and Regulatory Compliance 35

2.9 Measuring Administrative Efficiency and Performance 36
KPIs and Benchmarking 36
Feedback 37
Lean Six Sigma 37

2.10 Practice in Action 37

2.11 Summary 38

Chapter 3: Staffing and Operations 41

3.1 Introduction 41

3.2 Key Financial and Operational Staffing Indicators 42
Navigating Staffing Efficiency and Effectiveness 42
Utilizing Staffing Indicators for Strategic Management 44
Future Trends: Predictive Analytics in Staffing 44

3.3 Optimizing Staffing Models in Healthcare 45
    Types of Staffing Models 46
    Key Considerations When Selecting Staffing Models 48

3.4 Recruitment and Retention 50
    Recruitment Strategies 51
    Retention Strategies 53
    Engagement Strategies 55

3.5 Strategic Outsourcing and Automation in Healthcare 57
    Evaluation of Areas for Outsourcing and/or Automation 58
    Outsourcing Models 59
    Automation 60

3.6 Diversity, Equity and Inclusion in Healthcare Leadership 63
    Importance of DEI in Healthcare 63
    Strategies for Promoting DEI 64
    Leadership's Role in DEI 65

3.7 Understanding Labor Law for Operational Leaders 65
    Wage and Hour Laws 65
    Anti-Discrimination Laws 67
    Occupational Safety and Health Act (OSHA) 69

3.8 Practice in Action 69

3.9 Summary 71

Chapter 4: Current and Emerging Physicians Models 75

4.1 Introduction 75

4.2 Challenges of Physician Engagement and Retention 76

4.3 Employed Physician Model 78
    Advantages 79
    Challenges 80

4.4 Engaging and Retaining Employed Physicians 81
    Communication is Key 82
    Strategies for Physician Engagement, Retention and Wellness ... 82

4.5 Independent Physicians 84

4.6 Independent Practice Associations (IPAs) 89

4.7 Emerging Models for Physicians...91
   Remote Work Model 91
   Telehealth Model 92

4.8 Practice in Action...94

4.9 Summary 95

Chapter 5: Strategies for Physician Workplace Management 99

5.1 Introduction...99

5.2 Physician Retention Challenges and Impacts......................100
   Aging Physician Workforce 100
   Physician Shortages 101
   Physician Burnout 103

5.3 Physician Turnover Cost and Disruption............................105

5.4 KPIs: Measuring Retention, Burnout, and Turnover 107

5.5 Generational Differences in the Physician Workforce 110

5.6 Physician Compensation 112

5.7 Practice in Action... 114

5.8 Summary 115

Chapter 6: Financial Models and Revenue Cycle Management Functions.. 119

6.1 Introduction... 119

6.2 Care Delivery & Financial Models..120
   The Traditional Model: Fee for Service 121
   A Newer Model: Value-Based Care... 121
   A Refreshed Model: Population-Based Payments.....................122
   The Disruptor Model: Private Pay and Concierge 123
   Partnership Model: Independent Medical Practices
      and Larger Hospitals...123

6.3 Functions Within Care Delivery Models 124
  Revenue Cycle Management (RCM) 124
  Contracting (also known as Managed Care Contracting) 125
  Pre-visit Activities 125
  Registration Activities 126
  Charting 126
  Claims Processing 127
  Denial Management 127
  Payments and Receivables Management 128
  Post Audit and Process Improvement 129

6.4 Key Performance Indicators 129

6.5 Practice in Action 130

6.6 Summary 131

Chapter 7: Payer Contracting 135

7.1 Introduction 135

7.2 Review Contract Performance 136

7.3 Compare Contract Performance 139

7.4 Define Payer Targets and Proposals 141
  Proposal Preparation 145

7.5 Deploy Negotiation Communication Plan 147
  Value Proposition 147

7.6 Evaluate Proposals/Counters 150

7.7 Negotiate Language/Execute Agreement 151
  Rates 152
  Term 152
  Termination 153
  Penalties 153

7.8 Practice in Action 154

7.9 Summary 155

Chapter 8: The Data Scene 157

    8.1 Introduction 157
           Digging into Data 158

    8.2 Data Sources and Collection 160
           Internal sources of financial and performance data 160
           External Sources of Data 164

    8.3 Utilizing Data 167
           Standardizing Data to Create Comparison Metrics 167

    8.4 Key Performance Indicators (KPIs) 168
           Identifying Measures of Healthcare Quality 171

    8.5 Benchmarking Concepts 172
           History of Benchmarking 173
           Benefits of Benchmarking 173
           Types of Benchmarking 174
           Other Benchmarking Terminology 175
           Describing the Benchmarking Process 175
           Why Your Organization Needs Benchmarking 177

    8.6 Process Benchmarking 178
           The Benefits of Process Benchmarking: 180
           Peer Networks and Management Collaboratives 181
           Benchmarking Quality 183

    8.7 Practice in Action 186

    8.8 Summary 187

Chapter 9: Marketing Strategies for Medical Practices 191

    9.1 Introduction 191

    9.2 The Importance of Healthcare Marketing Strategy 192
           Unique Challenges and Considerations in Healthcare
               Marketing 194

    9.3 Understanding Your Target Audience 195
           Conducting Effective Market Research 195
           Analyzing Market Trends and Competition 197

9.4 Developing a Strong Brand Identity 198
    Crafting a Compelling Brand 199
    Developing a Unique Value Proposition 199
    Designing a Professional and Visually Appealing Brand
        Identity 200

9.5 Online Presence and Your Website 201
    Building an Effective Website 202
    How to Do Content Marketing 203
    How Long Until You See Growth? 205

9.6 Patient Referral Programs and Relationship Management 205
    Building Relationships with Referring Physicians
        and Healthcare Professionals 206
    Enhancing Patient Experience and Satisfaction 206
    Implementing a Patient Referral Program 207

9.7 Community Engagement and Local Marketing 207
    Strategies for Effective Community Engagement 208

9.8 Patient Testimonials and Online Reviews 209
    How to Address Negative Feedback 209

9.9 Measuring and Analyzing Marketing Performance 211
    Setting Marketing Goals 211
    Identifying the Marketing KPIs of Your Practice 211
    Analyzing Marketing Performance 212

9.10 What's Next & Future Trends in Healthcare Marketing 213
    Adapting to Technological Innovations 214
    Embracing Digital Transformation 215
    Sustainability and Social Responsibility 215

9.11 Practice in Action 216

9.12 Summary 219

Chapter 10: Advanced Health IT Strategies for Medical Practices 221

10.1 Introduction 221

10.2 Electronic Health Records (EHR) 222
  User Interface and Usability 223
  Time Consuming Data Entry 224
  Interoperability Issues 225

10.3 Health Information Exchange 226
  What is HIE? 227
  Benefits of HIE 227
  Challenges of Health Information Exchange 228
  Legal and Privacy Issues in Health Information Exchange 228

10.4 Telemedicine, RPM and RTM 229
  The Growing Importance of Telemedicine and RPM 230
  Strategies for Integrating Telemedicine 231
  Leveraging RPM Technologies for Improved Patient Outcomes 233
  Overcoming Barriers and Maximizing Benefits of Telemedicine 236

10.5 Patient Engagement and Health Apps 237
  Engaging Patients through Digital Platforms 238
  Evaluating and Integrating Health Apps into Medical Practices 238
  Ensuring Data Security in Patient Engagement Technologies 240

10.6 Cybersecurity and Data Privacy in Medical Practices 240
  Cybersecurity Threats Faced by Medical Practices 241
  Ensuring Data Security and Privacy in EHR Usage 242
  Implementing Robust Security Measures to Protect Patient Data ... 243
  Complying with Data Privacy Regulations and Ensuring Ethical Data Use 243
  Training Staff on Cybersecurity Awareness and Best Practices ... 244

10.7 Future Outlook 245

10.8 Practice in Action 246

10.9 Summary 247

Chapter 11: Managing Risk and Compliance in a Medical Practice 251

11.1 Introduction 251

11.2 Identifying and Assessing Risks 252
   Clinical Risks 252
   Operational Risks..253
   Financial Risks 254
   Legal Risks..255
   Establishing a Risk Management Framework Assessment 256
   Prioritizing Risks...258
   Other Tools and Frameworks for Risk Analysis 259

11.3 Developing Risk Management Strategies 263
   Establishing Policies, Procedures and Protocols to Mitigate
      Risks..268
   Implementing Patient Safety Initiatives....................................270
   Challenges in Adopting Patient Safety Practices........................270
   Ensuring Compliance with Regulatory Requirements
      and Legal Considerations 274

11.4 Incident Response...275
   Building a Culture of Safety and Encouraging Error
      Reporting..275
   Establishing Incident Response Protocols and Procedures 276

11.5 Communication and Documentation 277
   Ensuring Clear and Concise Documentation..........................278
   Educating Staff on Risk Awareness...279

11.6 Monitoring and Evaluation...280
   Collecting and Analyzing Data...280
   Incorporating Feedback and Lessons Learned.........................281

11.7 Practice in Action 282

11.8 Summary 283

Conclusion 287

Index 289

Chapter 11: Managing Risk and Compliance in a Medical
Practice..251

11.1 Introduction..251

11.2 Identifying and Assessing Risks...252
   Clinical Risks...252
   Operational Risks..253
   Financial Risks..254
   Legal Risks..255
   Establishing a Risk Management Framework Framework..257
   Monitoring Risks...258
   Other Tools and Frameworks for Risk Analysis..................259

11.3 Developing Risk Management Strategies..........................265
   Establishing Policies, Procedures and Protocols to Mitigate
   Risks..268
   Implementing Patient Safety Measures...............................270
   Challenges in Mitigating Risk in Safety Incidents..............270
   Ensuring Compliance with Regulatory Requirements
   and Accreditation Standards..274

11.4 Incident Response..277
   Building a Culture of Safety and Encouraging Error
   Reporting..278
   Establishing Clear Roles, Protocols, and Procedures..........278

11.5 Communication and Documentation................................279
   Creating Clear and Effective Documentation....................279
   Effective Risk Communication...279

11.6 Monitoring and Evaluation..280
   Monitoring and Reporting..281
   Continuous Feedback and Improvement...........................281

11.7 Practical Application..282

11.8 Summary...283

Conclusion..285

Index..289

Contributors

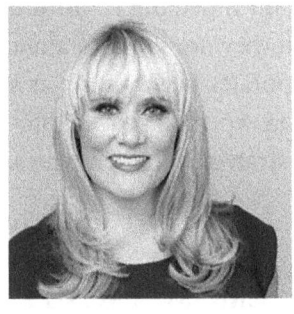

Dawn Plested, FACHE, MBA, JD, ESQ., has an extensive background in healthcare management and consulting. She has experience in operations leadership, Value-Based Purchasing arrangements and innovative payment models, strategic planning, risk and compliance, marketing and communications, employee and physician engagement and management, and policy and procedure development. She has worked with private practices, hospital-based systems, rural health clinics and FQHCs. Dawn has an MBA with an emphasis in healthcare and international leadership as well as a Juris Doctorate (JD) with a health law emphasis. Licensed to practice law in Minnesota, Dawn is also trained in Alternative Dispute Resolution as a mediator and arbitrator. With over 15 years of experience in a variety of healthcare leadership roles, Dawn has a unique skill set thanks to her education combined with broad experience in operations, finance, policy, leadership, marketing, communications and public relations. This skill set makes her uniquely qualified to provide expertise in a consulting role.

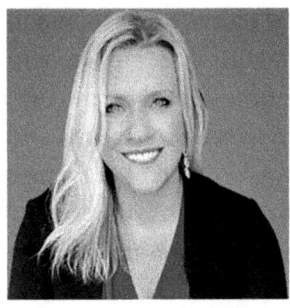

Adrienne Lloyd, MHA, FACHE, helps healthcare leaders and practice owners build top-tier organizations with empowered teams and optimized processes so they can reduce burnout and scale to serve more patients while achieving their personal and professional goals. Adrienne has worked as a healthcare executive for over 20 years, including 10 years at Mayo Clinic in chief executive and director-level roles along with seven years at Duke Health System as the chief administrative officer for Duke Ophthalmology and Surgical Practices. She spent most of her career helping improve organizations while driving integrations and building teams that worked together to improve the patient and organizational experience. Thanks to these initiatives, she has helped generate more than $250 million in financial, patient care and team improvements. Adrienne founded Optimize Healthcare to help other healthcare executives and physician leaders reshape their organizations. Her signature Day Zero Blueprint™ program is helping transform leaders and organizations as they shift the belief that they need to do it alone or sacrifice what is important to them. She incorporates her training as a John Maxwell Certified Coach and Lean/Six Sigma expert to provide program participants and audiences with time-saving strategies and templates.

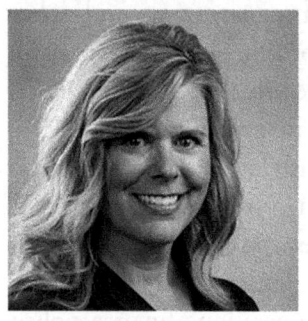

Jessica Minesinger, CMOM, FACMPE, is the Founder and CEO of Surgical Compensation & Consulting (SCC), working with physicians to navigate compensation opportunities. Using data analytics, she empowers physicians to negotiate successfully, ensure pay equality and identify cultural fit. Jessica is an entrepreneur at heart, a problem-solver, and a firm believer in the power of data and analytics. She is a Fellow of the American College of Medical Practice Executives (ACMPE), a member of the American Association of Provider Compensation Professionals (AAPCP), and an Affiliate Member of the American College of Surgeons and the Association of Women Surgeons. With an extensive background in surgical practice development, management, physician contracting, compensation analysis, and human resources, Jessica has a deep understanding of the unique and often complex nature of the business side of medicine. After running a trauma and acute care surgery practice for 10 years, Jessica was inspired to leverage her knowledge and expertise to help physicians and surgeons successfully navigate compensation opportunities and negotiate their value through every stage of their careers.

Contributors

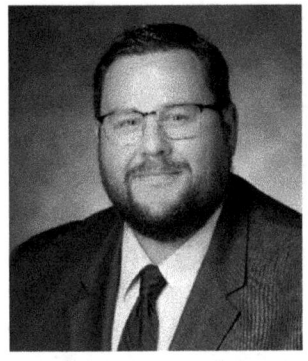

Jonathan Leer, CHFP, CMPE, has over 14 years of healthcare administration and healthcare finance experience in for-profit healthcare, not-for-profit systems, consulting and academic medical centers. Joining Johns Hopkins University in 2022 as the Division Administrator of Geriatric Medicine and Gerontology, Jonathan is a Fellow of the Healthcare Financial Management Association and a Fellow of the American College of Medical Practice Executives, with both certifications being the highest achievement bestowed in either organization. Jonathan is also an active member of the American College of Healthcare Executives and has spoken at numerous national conferences on the topics of physician management and education of business concepts to healthcare providers. Originally from Fort Smith, Ark., Jonathan earned a bachelor's degree in Business Administration and double majored in Accounting and Finance at Texas Christian University. He then earned master's degrees in accounting and healthcare administration from the University of Texas system, where he later taught health finance and accounting as an adjunct professor in their CAHME-accredited MHA program. Prior to joining Johns Hopkins Medicine, Jonathan worked at UT Southwestern Medical Center for the Department of Pediatrics in multiple management roles.

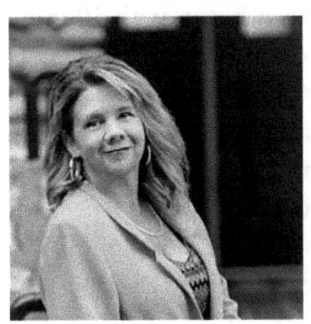

Doral Davis-Jacobsen, MBA, FACMPE, is a managing consultant with over 20 years of experience in healthcare business process improvement, focusing on next-generation managed care contracting, revenue cycle benchmarking, operations optimization, quality initiatives, financial modeling and project management. Doral has experience managing clinics and billing operations for large practices on the provider side, while negotiating contracts and working with a management company administering risk products in an IPA environment on the payer side. As a healthcare advisor, Doral successfully worked with a large medical practice on revenue cycle efficiency and benchmarking to improve collections by $2.8 million in less than a year. She also worked with a small medical practice on revenue cycle optimization and improved physician compensation by 35% within two years. She even piloted the first Real-Time Claim Adjudication project utilizing front-end processes, which received wide publicity from multiple publications, including *Modern Healthcare*, *Radiology Today* and *The Journal of Medical Practice Management*. Doral has authored numerous articles and co-authored the 2016 MGMA book *Transitioning to Alternative Payment Models: A Guide to Next Generation Managed Care Contracting* with fellow consultant Nanci Robertson.

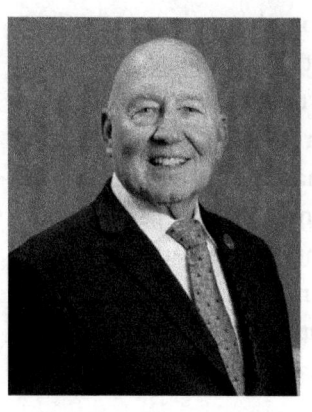

David N. Gans, MSHA, FACMPE served 42 years with MGMA as a Project Manager for federal and foundation grants, Director of Survey Operations, Vice President of Research and Innovation and Senior Fellow, Industry Affairs. Since retiring in early 2022, he remains an active volunteer, serving as an educational speaker and authoring the Data Mine column for the *MGMA Connection*. David has also been a Member of the Board of Directors for the Accreditation Association for Ambulatory Health Care (AAAHC) since 2020. David's career began with 10 years active duty in the U.S. Army Medical Service Corps, followed by 21 years of service in the U.S. Army Reserve, retiring in the rank of Colonel. He received his Bachelor of Arts degree in Government from the University of Notre Dame and has a Master of Science in Education degree from the University of Southern California, along with a Master of Science in Health Administration degree from the University of Colorado. He is a Certified Medical Practice Executive and a Life Fellow in the American College of Medical Practice Executives.

Contributors

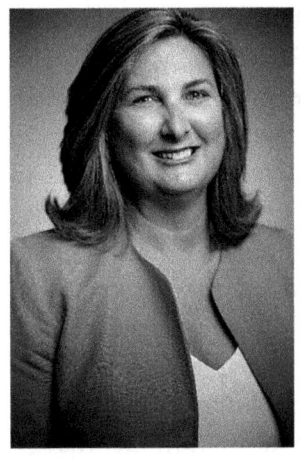

Jennifer Thompson, MHA, has served as President of Insight Marketing Group since 2006 and helps physicians and private medical practices throughout the U.S. attract and retain patients and rock-star employees. Jennifer has over 20 years of experience in marketing and business development for start-up organizations and as a marketing director for a Fortune 500 company. She is the co-founder and chief strategist for Dr Marketing Tips Lab, a website designed to help medical marketing professionals. Jennifer is also a former elected official, serving as County Commissioner in Orange County Florida from 2011-2018. During her two terms, she served as a member of the Central Florida Expressway Authority (CFX), Central Florida Research Park and the Orange County Arts & Cultural Affairs Committee. Jennifer holds a master's degree in Healthcare Administration from the University of Central Florida.

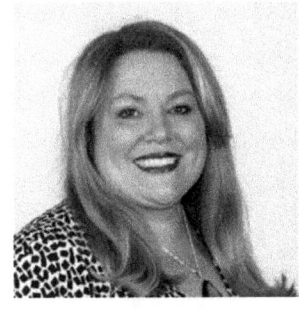

Katie Nunn, MBA, CMPE, provides training and coaching for healthcare leaders and their organizations on process improvement, financial optimization and cultural transformation. Leveraging extensive experience with financial and operational turnarounds, she is a valuable advisor for an organization experiencing rapid expansion or change. With over 20 years of experience in healthcare leadership, her broad areas of expertise include practice assessments, process improvement, financial management, IT implementations, telemedicine, strategic planning, provider on-boarding and cultural transformation. From 2008-2019, Katie served as the Chief Administrator for Pulmonary Associates of Richmond, one of the nation's largest private pulmonary practices with 32 physicians and 22 Advanced Practice Clinicians. Over her 11 years at PAR, Katie drove substantial change that resulted in a 300% increase in revenue and a 32% increase in shareholder income while increasing employee and patient satisfaction.

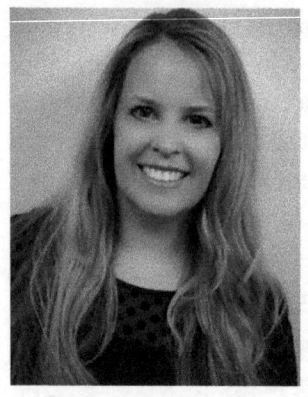

Cristy Good, MPH, MBA, CPC, CMPE, is a Senior Industry Advisor at MGMA, with expertise in practice management, healthcare operations, revenue cycle management and project management. She has more than 20 years of experience in medical practice administration and financial management. Prior to joining MGMA, Cristy was a credentialed trainer with EPIC and helped prepare providers for one of the largest EHR implementations. For more than five years, she was an administrator with a large health system where she oversaw the strategic and daily operations for multiple outpatient medical practices and also spent six months working for a private home health agency. In addition, she has more than 10 years of clinical laboratory experience.

Introduction

This is the third book in MGMA's *Advanced Strategy for Medical Practice Leaders* series. Volume one was the *Financial Management Edition*, and covered best financial practices that can help optimize revenue cycle integrity and minimize costs for healthcare organizations. Volume two, the *Human Resources Management Edition*, looked at how modern medical group practices can integrate human resource strategies to improve the employment lifecycle and organizational culture. This *Operations Management Edition* will conclude this series as it explores the key aspects of overall administrative operations and structures for medical practices.

This *Operations Management Edition* provides a comprehensive guide to advanced and yet critical components of effective operations management in medical practices. It serves as a valuable resource for healthcare leaders and administrators seeking to enhance their organization's efficiency, productivity and provide high quality patient centric care delivery.

The book begins by reviewing the foundational elements of any successful medical practice, which is the mission, vision and values. Understanding how to align these guiding principles while engaging key stakeholders and maintaining a culture of operational excellence and quality improvement is essential. We then will examine the various administrative structures and leadership approaches that strengthen efficient practice operations. This includes topics such as organizational design, implementation of health information systems and actionable strategies for optimizing staffing and scheduling.

A large portion of this book is dedicated to the financial and operational aspects of running a high-performing best in class medical practice.

We will explore the landscape of various delivery models, from traditional fee-for-service to value-based or other population health-based approaches. Mastering revenue cycle management, payer contracting and data analytics are also covered due to the critical relationship they have with financial sustainability. The book also dives into marketing strategies, the effective use of technology and risk management—all of which are increasingly important in today's environment which is seemingly changing by the hour.

Throughout the book, we have included real-world examples from experienced healthcare experts. These first-hand accounts provide valuable context and demonstrate how these strategies and concepts can be applied within various medical practice settings. Whether you are part of a large health organization or a small, independent practice, the principles outlined in this resource will be relevant to your unique organizational needs.

This book will empower healthcare leaders of today and tomorrow to drive meaningful change and enhance organizational performance—ultimately with the goal to deliver the highest quality patient care. As the final edition of the *Advanced Strategy for Medical Practice Leaders* series, this *Operations Management Edition* will prepare you with the knowledge and tools necessary to lead your practice successfully into the future with confidence.

Chapter 1

Defining the Heart of your Organization

By: Adrienne Palmer Lloyd,
MHA, FACHE

1.1 Introduction

In healthcare, operational leadership hinges on the robust foundation of an organization's mission, vision and values. These elements are vital, shaping not only the strategic direction but also the day-to-day operational decisions that impact patient care and employee engagement. They not only articulate the organization's core purpose and promises to the community while providing a roadmap of the desired future, but they also define the ethical and moral compass of the organization, ensuring that all actions align with its overarching principles. Together, these elements form the bedrock of a healthcare organization, driving it to fulfill its purpose and make a lasting, positive impact on patients and the community. This chapter will discuss how to set the tone for effective and ethical operational management within your healthcare organization.

1.2 Mission, Vision and Values

Operational leadership in healthcare is fundamentally grounded in the organization's mission, vision and values. Ensuring you create and implement these core elements can help set the tone for all staffing and operational decisions, and develop alignment with the organization's overarching principles. They are not merely words on a page but a reflection of the organization's soul, shaping its identity and serving as the North Star for all its endeavors.

Mission Statement

A mission statement is the soul of a healthcare organization and should articulate your core purpose. In healthcare, it is the promise to the community served and a declaration of the impact it intends to make on the lives of patients. It encapsulates why your organization exists, what it aims to achieve and for whom. It is the driving force behind every action taken by the organization.

A well-crafted mission statement inspires and rallies everyone involved, from the executive leadership to the frontline healthcare workers, around a common purpose. The statement should be clear and memorable, ensuring that everyone within your organization can easily articulate it.

For example, the Mayo Clinic declares its mission as "To inspire hope and contribute to health and well-being by providing the best care to every patient through integrated clinical practice, education and research."[1] This mission is a testament to their commitment to not just healing patients but also advancing medical knowledge through research and education.

Vision Statement

The vision statement paints a clear picture of the future your healthcare organization aspires to create. It should be inspirational, motivating and forward-thinking. A compelling vision statement serves as a guiding principle for your organization and motivates everyone involved to work toward a shared, ambitious goal. Leaders must ensure that the vision statement is aligned with the mission and values, creating a cohesive narrative that drives the organization forward. The vision statement builds on the foundations of the mission statement by communicating your future aspirations and sets a path to the future.[2]

Chapter 1: Defining the Heart of your Organization

Values

Values represent the core beliefs and principles that guide the behavior and decisions of individuals within the organization. They are the ethical and moral compass that ensures actions align with the organization's mission and vision. Values set the tone for the organizational culture. They define the behaviors and principles that are non-negotiable. These values should resonate with your team and stakeholders.

Leaders must not only articulate these values but also demonstrate them through their actions. A values-driven culture fosters trust, collaboration and ethical decision-making, which are essential in the healthcare sector.

In a healthcare setting, values often relate to compassion, integrity, accountability and a commitment to patient-centered care. For instance, the Cleveland Clinic outlines its values as "Caring for life, researching for health, educating those who serve."[3] These values are not merely slogans but are deeply ingrained in the organization's DNA, and are reflected in the way they care for patients and engage with their teams.

Mayo Clinic founder Dr. William J. Mayo suggested that three conditions were essential for his organization's future success:[4]

1. The continuing pursuit of the ideal of service over profit;
2. Primary concern for the care and welfare of each patient; and
3. The continuing interest by every member of the organization in the professional progress of every other member.

That philosophy has in turn helped establish the clinic's vision and values, with a culture shaped by both explicit and implicit displays of how those values are embraced and used to make day-to-day decisions. As described in an MGMA article about the impact of those values on organizational success, "members of the Mayo Clinic staff embrace and reinforce the primary value and regard it as a professionalism covenant: a collective, tacit agreement that everyone will earnestly collaborate to put the needs and welfare of patients first."[5]

The clinic has long established a Values Council to reflect upon those values and see that they are put in action by all employees, which includes presentations to groups across the entire clinic system, as well as financial support for values-based research and quality improvement projects. The Mayo Clinic values are also included in HR functions including orientation, performance evaluations and 360-degree feedback.

MVV Sets the Tone for Your Organization's Success

The triad of mission, vision and values is the cornerstone of operational leadership in healthcare. A well-defined mission and vision, coupled with strong core values, not only provide clarity and purpose but also foster a culture of shared dedication to the well-being of patients and the communities that healthcare organizations serve.

Here are the reasons why these concepts are so crucial in the world of healthcare leadership:

- **Clarity of Purpose:** A well-crafted mission statement provides clarity of purpose. It helps leaders and team members understand the "why" behind what they do. In healthcare, where every action can impact patient outcomes, knowing the purpose is grounding.
- **Goal Alignment:** A clear vision statement aligns everyone within the organization toward common goals. It sets the direction for the future, serving as a unifying force that keeps all efforts moving in the same direction.
- **Culture Building:** Values, when consistently upheld, build the culture of the organization. They define the expectations for behavior, ethics and decision-making. In healthcare, where ethical considerations are paramount, values guide actions and foster a culture of trust and integrity.

How to Align MVV with Your Organization's Goals

Aligning your mission, vision and values with your organization's goals is a process that requires thoughtful consideration and intentional effort.

Chapter 1: Defining the Heart of your Organization

If these are already in place for your organization, it is good practice to assess them every few years to make sure they still represent your purpose, core values and direction. If these are not yet in place, spend time with both your leadership team and members of your physician and employee teams to obtain input into what you truly value and want to build towards. According to Forbes contributor Kathy Miller Perkins, PhD, this will require you to regularly check in with employees. You can also observe their behavior in employee events and directly discuss how people interpret your company's values, to see if those goals need to be refined.[6]

Here are steps to help you align and implement these core components:

1. Reflect on Your Core Purpose: Begin by reflecting on the core purpose of your healthcare organization by considering the following:

- Why does it exist?
- What does it aim to achieve for patients and the community it serves? Your mission should encapsulate this purpose succinctly.

2. Envision the Future: Craft a vision statement that envisions the future you want to create in healthcare.

- What does success look like in the long term?
- What transformative impact do you want to have on patient care, community health or the healthcare industry as a whole?

3. Define Your Values: Identify the values that underpin your healthcare organization's culture. These values should reflect the principles and ethics that guide your actions and serve as a moral compass for your team.

4. Ensure Consistency: It's not enough to have a well-crafted MVV; you must ensure consistency. Every decision, every action and every policy should be evaluated against your MVV. If they do not align, they should be reconsidered or adapted to maintain alignment.

Going through this process with your team can be a great opportunity to increase engagement and the sense of shared purpose across the organization, so please do not feel you have to navigate this alone.

5

The Vital Role of Consistency in Cultivating Culture

Consistency in culture is where the true potency of mission, vision and values emerges. They should not be mere words; they must be deeply ingrained in the fabric of your organization. According to Farhad Heidari, PhD, a culture of consistency emphasizes stability, routine and adherence to established processes and procedures, with a focus on maintaining standards and meeting expectations.[7]

Here's why consistency is indispensable:

- **Alignment of Efforts:** Consistency ensures that everyone within your healthcare organization is working in concert toward common objectives. It minimizes confusion and misdirection, facilitating efficient and coordinated efforts.
- **Trust and Predictability:** In healthcare, where trust is paramount, consistency in values and actions builds trust among patients, staff and stakeholders. When individuals can predict how your organization will respond in various situations, trust flourishes.
- **Culture Reinforcement:** Consistency in living out values reinforces the desired culture. It sets the standard for behavior and decision-making, offering guidance for everyone within the organization.

As Heidari notes, consistency must also be coupled with a culture of motivation, which provides the opportunity for personal growth and the development of more abstract qualities including purpose and autonomy. This can lead to improved employee engagement and satisfaction, and build more resilient workers.

Mission, vision and values are not merely abstract concepts; they constitute the essence of your healthcare organization. They define its purpose, direction and culture. Aligning them with organizational goals and ensuring their consistent application is paramount for success in healthcare leadership. These guiding principles serve as the foundation upon which you can construct a healthcare organization that not only fulfills its mission but also leaves a lasting, positive impact on patients and the community it serves.

1.3 Identifying and Engaging Key Players to Achieve Success

Effective leadership in healthcare requires collaboration that relies not only on one's individual capabilities but also the ability to understand, engage and synergize with a broad spectrum of stakeholders. Understanding their roles and fostering strong relationships is essential for success. Here are some of the key players you need to consider throughout your leadership career.

Physicians and Clinicians

Physicians and clinicians are at the heart of healthcare delivery. Building trust and collaboration with them is crucial for achieving clinical excellence. Leaders must recognize that physicians and clinicians bring unique expertise to patient care and effective communication, and partnerships with them are essential for providing high-quality healthcare services. According to the American Medical Association, physician-led, team-based care makes the best use of a physician's leadership knowledge, skills and expertise, identifying and engaging the proper contributions of other team members.[8] Regular meetings, interdisciplinary rounds and feedback mechanisms can facilitate collaboration and integrate clinical insights into the broader organizational strategy.

Nurses and Allied Health Professionals

Nurses and allied health professionals play critical roles in delivering patient care. Leaders should prioritize their well-being, professional growth and engagement. Creating a supportive work environment, offering opportunities for education and advancement, and involving them in decision-making processes are key strategies for retaining and empowering these crucial team members. The results can help promote the goals of safer and higher-quality care, as well as lower rates of burnout and employee turnover.[9]

Administrative and Support Staff

Administrative and support staff play critical roles in managing the operations of healthcare organizations. Effective leadership involves empowering and engaging these teams. Administrative and support staff are the backbone of healthcare organizations, managing front-line and behind the scenes patient flow, administrative tasks, billing and finance, data analytics, facility maintenance and logistics. Leaders should foster a culture of respect and appreciation for these roles by building open channels of communication. Empowering these teams to streamline processes and enhance efficiency can contribute significantly to overall organizational success.

Patients and Families

Healthcare leaders should engage patients and their families as partners in care. Their insights and feedback can drive improvements in patient experience. According to the Agency for Healthcare Research and Quality, patient engagement can also promote measurable improvements in safety and quality.[10] Patient and family engagement is a fundamental aspect of patient-centered care. Leaders should encourage open communication, actively seek patient feedback, and involve patients and families in decision-making processes when appropriate. Patient advisory councils and surveys are valuable tools for gathering insights and enhancing the patient experience.

Governing boards and Executive Committees

Lastly, the governance structure itself, including committees and boards, demands astute engagement. Executive leaders should work hand-in-hand with these bodies, aligning strategic initiatives with the overarching mission of the organization. Through transparent communication and shared governance models, executive leadership can drive accountability, innovation and strategic foresight across the healthcare landscape.

Engaging Key Stakeholders During Change

While consistently engaging your stakeholders through intentional feedback gathering, involvement in committees and initiatives and key

Chapter 1: Defining the Heart of your Organization

communication strategies is important. One of the most crucial times to do so is during times of change.

The SIPOC (Suppliers, Inputs, Process, Outputs, Customers) tool is a structure that you can use to identify key stakeholders in any process improvement, strategic, or change initiative.[11] This tool helps map out the suppliers, the inputs (who is involved in obtaining or creating them), the processes (who they may touch), the outputs and the end customers.

Exhibit 1.1 SIPOC Tool for Identifying Customers

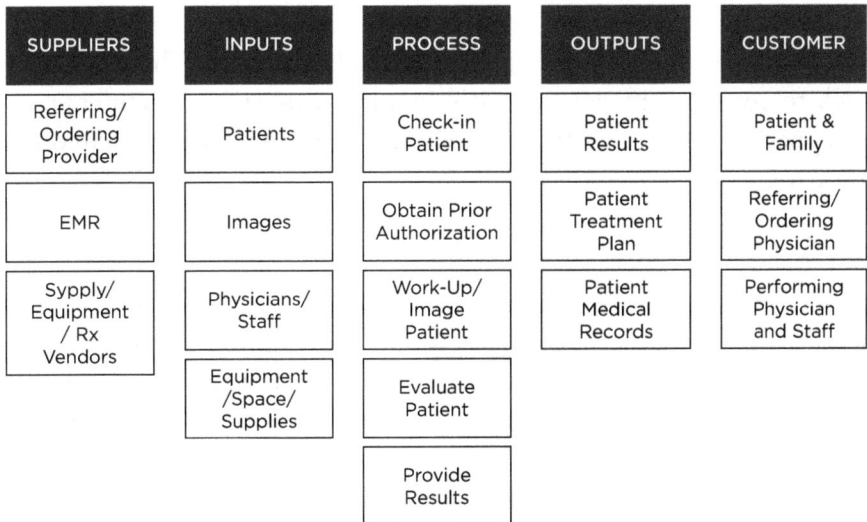

Taking the time to think through who is involved in each of these areas can identify who needs to be engaged and at what level. This can help you both gain additional input and better anticipate concerns or goals that need to be factored in during the change. By understanding and engaging your stakeholders, you will be better positioned as a healthcare leader to build alignment and drive results in a more seamless way.

The unifying thread through all these engagements is intentional, strategic leadership that understands the unique contributions of each role and seeks to unify them towards a common goal. This is not just about managing but about transforming the healthcare landscape through collaborative excellence.

9

1.4 Operational Excellence and Quality Improvement

In the dynamic landscape of healthcare, operational excellence and quality improvement are not just ideals to strive for; they are essential components for success and sustainability. Integrating these as core approaches not only improves outcomes and efficiency but provides tools to enhance collaboration, input and partnership across teams to ultimately foster a culture that prioritizes continuous innovation.

Lean and Six Sigma in Healthcare

Lean and Six Sigma, both derived from manufacturing principles, have found significant applications in healthcare.[12] These concepts seek to combine efficiencies with ongoing process improvements, all designed to streamline healthcare operations and improve outcomes for patients.

Lean

Lean focuses on eliminating waste (non-value-added activities), optimizing processes and maximizing value. Healthcare leaders can apply Lean thinking to streamline workflows, reduce wait times and enhance patient experiences. It involves continuous improvement by examining processes and removing inefficiencies, such as unnecessary steps in patient admissions or excessive inventory levels.

Value under Lean is always defined from the perspective of the ***customer*** and is looking at what the customer would be willing to pay for. Unfortunately, a lot of what is done in healthcare, some due to regulatory and billing requirements and some due to inefficiencies, is not really value-added from the perspective of the patients. The good news is that this affords the opportunity to really evaluate whether to take that next step or if there is a better way to achieve the same outcome with less time and/or fewer resources.

Lean principles go beyond cost reduction; they are about delivering value to patients efficiently. Leaders should champion Lean principles across the organization, encouraging teams to identify and eliminate waste in their daily processes. This may involve conducting value stream mapping, creating standardized work procedures and fostering a culture of continuous improvement.

Six Sigma

Six Sigma is a data-driven approach to process improvement that emphasizes reducing variability and defects in processes. In healthcare, Six Sigma principles can be applied to reduce medical errors, enhance patient safety and optimize clinical processes. Implementing Six Sigma involves defining problems, measuring current performance, analyzing root causes, improving processes and continuously monitoring results.

Lean vs. Six Sigma

It's essential for healthcare leaders to understand the distinctions between Lean and Six Sigma. While both methodologies focus on process improvement, they have distinct differences in areas of emphasis. Lean, as mentioned earlier, centers on eliminating waste and optimizing value delivery to patients. In contrast, Six Sigma is primarily concerned with reducing process variation and minimizing defects. Lean often starts by identifying waste and seeks to streamline processes by eliminating unnecessary steps and reducing cycle times. Six Sigma, on the other hand, begins with identifying process variation and aims to minimize it by using statistical analysis and problem-solving tools. The combination of Lean and Six Sigma, often referred to as Lean Six Sigma, brings together the strengths of both methodologies to create a comprehensive approach to process improvement in healthcare organizations.

Because of the immense amount of waste in healthcare, it's recommended to utilize Lean tools first to map the process and identify steps or components that can be stopped. By doing so you do not spend time perfecting the training or editing the form when there may be a way to eliminate that step in the first place and still improve the overall process.

Process Improvement Tools

Here are a core set of process improvement tools and strategies leaders can incorporate individually or as a large-scale improvement effort to identify, analyze and implement changes:

Brainstorming: A collaborative and dedicated session of idea generation, brainstorming is designed to encourage the thoughts and possible solutions of those directly involved in the work at hand. Brainstorming focuses on quality and is open to all ideas to help make process improvements.

Current/Future/Ideal Value Stream Maps: The VSM helps identify the actions necessary to bring service to either patients or payees. It is a process map that allows you to see and understand the flow of objects, patients, materials, supplies and information through a clinic's daily processes.[13] It can be useful in reducing cycle time. Future or ideal workflow models can help build efficiency and set priorities.

5S Waste Walk and Standard Work: Adapted from the manufacturing floor, a clean, safe and well-organized workspace is exemplified in five steps: "sort, set in order, shine, standardize and sustain." Physically examining the work environment and removing clutter and redundancy, as well as standardizing work processes, will help bring continuous improvement to processes.[14]

Spaghetti Mapping: A visual diagram of the flow of workers and products within the daily healthcare processes. It provides a description of where employees are physically moving within the workplace, which can help avoid unnecessary movement and processes.[15]

5 Whys: Repeatedly asking "why" when a problem is encountered in the workflow will help go beyond the obvious symptoms and uncover the root cause of the issue. Understanding the way that work is done by investigating the process can lead to better countermeasures.[16]

Time Observation/Data Analysis: Observing and recording the amount of time required to complete individual processes can provide objective and comprehensive feedback on various processes. These and other concrete pieces of workplace data can be analyzed to improve efficiency.

Chapter 1: Defining the Heart of your Organization

Exhibit 1.2 Process Improvement Toolkit

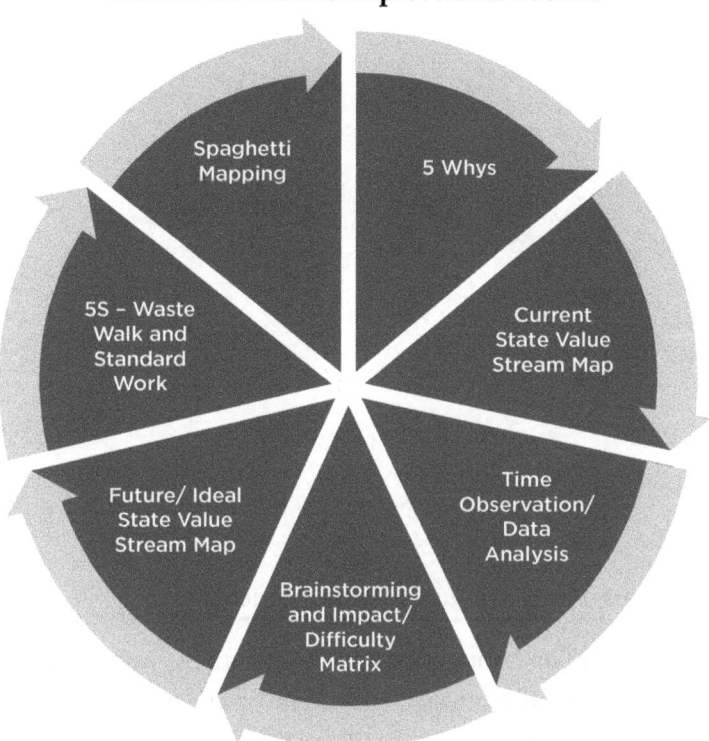

WEEDOUTS: Another straightforward way to begin process improvement is to begin looking for wastes across an individual process and then across the organization. The key categories of waste can be identified through the acronym "WEEDOUTS":

- **W**aiting: for testing, for physician, for team members, for results
- **E**xcess Motion: staff movement to finish testing
- **E**xcess Transportation: unnecessary patient movement
- **D**efects or Errors: poor work quality, scheduling errors
- **O**verproducing: producing service too early or frequently
- **U**nnecessary Processing: imaging that exceeds practice needs
- **T**oo much Material or Information: excess inventory, space
- **S**taffing: excess or wasted effort/time, inconsistent workloads

13

Exhibit 1.3 WEEDOUTS Chart

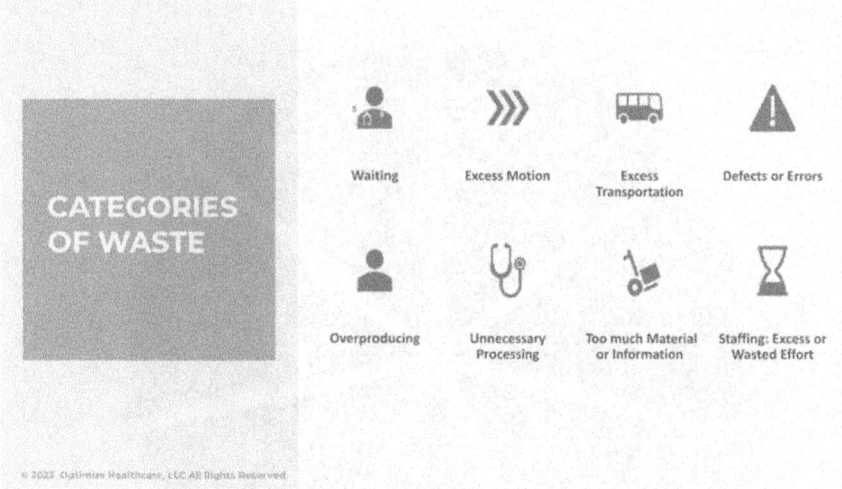

Engaging Your Team in Quality Improvement

The success of operational excellence and quality improvement initiatives heavily relies on the engagement and involvement of the entire healthcare team. As a leader, fostering a culture where every team member feels empowered to contribute to process improvements is crucial. This involves:

- **Training and Education:** Equip your team with the necessary knowledge and skills in Lean and Six Sigma methodologies.
- **Communication:** Maintain open lines of communication to understand challenges faced by staff and to share success stories.
- **Collaboration:** Encourage interdisciplinary collaboration to facilitate a comprehensive approach to quality improvement.

Engaging your team not only improves processes but also boosts morale and job satisfaction, leading to lower turnover rates.

The Virginia Mason Institute was a pioneer in utilizing Lean in healthcare and has resources around performing a "Waste Walk" with

Chapter 1: Defining the Heart of your Organization

your team, using a hands-on approach to discover and address waste in your organization.[17] This can be a great way to actively engage your team and create fast "visual" changes that allow momentum to build towards making larger improvements.

Remember, one of the most important steps of any process improvement is to create a deeper understanding of the workflows, metrics and goals across your teams so they are engaged in driving ongoing improvement throughout the organization.

MIPS and Quality Metrics

The Merit-based Incentive Payment System (MIPS) is a critical component in the U.S. healthcare system, influencing reimbursement and emphasizing quality of care.[18] MIPS measures performance in four areas: Quality, Cost, Improvement Activities and Promoting Interoperability. Healthcare leaders must understand these metrics and incorporate them into their quality improvement strategies.

Focusing on quality metrics under MIPS, such as patient outcomes, safety measures, and patient experience, aligns operational goals with federal standards. This not only ensures compliance but also drives improvements in patient care quality.

Cultivating a Culture of High-Quality Care

To ensure a culture of high-quality care, healthcare leaders must:

- **Utilize Data:** Before you can set changes in motion, you need to understand your current state for a given area or metric. It is beneficial to benchmark nationally or with other organizations and areas when possible to help illustrate the need for any changes and partner closely with your physicians and clinical teams to understand key drivers and implement changes.
- **Set Clear Goals:** Define clear, measurable goals for quality improvement. Use specific metrics to track progress.
- **Patient-Centric Approach:** Always prioritize patient needs and experiences in process improvement strategies.

- **Encourage Innovation:** Create an environment where staff are encouraged to come up with innovative solutions to improve quality.
- **Regular Reviews and Adjustments:** Continuously monitor processes and outcomes, making adjustments as necessary to maintain high standards of care.

1.5 Practice in Action

Recognizing the need to enhance the hospital's fulfillment of its mission as a religious organization, the chief executive officer of Lutheran Hospital of Indiana, Inc., Fort Wayne, initiated a process to change the institution's corporate culture to reflect the mission.

After assessing hospital managers' perceptions of the hospital's mission, a planning committee drafted a mission statement. The statement was condensed into a new motto which reflected the Lutheran organization's values and vision. The desire was to explicitly guide employees' actions in the spirit of doing the best for patients and families, at all times.

The hospital expanded its job descriptions to include the facility's expectations for employee behavior that is consistent with the mission. It also initiated an orientation program for new employees which emphasized incorporating the concepts of courtesy and compassion into all activities. To establish the mission firmly as part of the corporate culture, the hospital established three recognition programs and redesigned its pay plan to recognize performance that reflected the hospital's mission. The hospital facility was also redecorated, which helped improve employees' attitudes toward their work environment.

Five years into the change process, the hospital now has clear direction for strategic decisions, a more cooperative atmosphere and increased admissions. The process continues, and assessment of the mission establishment process will lead to the initiation of continuous quality improvement concepts.[19]

Chapter 1: Defining the Heart of your Organization

1.6 Summary

Operational excellence and quality improvement in healthcare are multifaceted and require a comprehensive approach. By effectively implementing Lean and Six Sigma methodologies, engaging your team, understanding and incorporating MIPS and quality metrics, and fostering a culture centered around high-quality care, healthcare leaders can significantly enhance patient outcomes and organizational performance. This journey towards excellence is continuous and requires dedication, innovation and a relentless focus on patient care quality.

To summarize, here are some of the key points discussed in this chapter:

- A well-articulated mission statement, vision statement and values can help set the tone for organizational success. They provide clarity of purpose, goal alignment and culture-building models that can be understood and implemented by employees at every level.
- Mission and vision statements as well as values should be aligned with organizational goals. This requires reflecting on core purpose, envisioning the future, defining those values and ensuring consistency.
- Consistency promotes trust and predictability, reinforces culture and aligns a team's efforts. It should also be coupled with a culture of motivation, which fosters purpose, autonomy and personal growth.
- Identify key players in the organization and engage with them on a regular basis, including physicians, nursing and health professionals, administrative and support staff, patients and their families, as well as governing boards and committees.
- Operational excellence and quality improvement strategies such as the manufacturing-derived Lean Six Sigma can be vital in creating a culture of continuous process improvement. Its tools can help identify waste and redundancy and empower employees to help guide changes. The Merit-based

17

Incentive Payment System (MIPS) and other quality metrics can be used to gauge their success.
- A culture of high-quality care can be cultivated by using data, setting clear goals, adopting a patient-centric approach, encouraging innovation and making regular reviews and adjustments, as necessary.

The next chapter will look at a variety of administrative structures which can help achieve these goals and mission by optimizing a medical practice' operations.

Notes

1. Mayo Clinic Health System. https://www.mayoclinichealthsystem.org/locations/red-wing/about-us/mission-vision-values
2. Leaders.com. https://leaders.com/articles/company-culture/vision-statement/
3. Cleveland Clinic. https://my.clevelandclinic.org/about/overview/who-we-are/mission-vision-values
4. Fleming RW. "The Mayo Culture." Mayo Foundation for Medical Education and Research, 1986.
5. MGMA. https://www.mgma.com/articles/the-impact-of-values-on-organizational-success
6. Forbes. https://www.forbes.com/sites/kathymillerperkins/2019/10/12/assessing-organizational-culture-made-simple/?sh=7e7bf78534cc
7. LinkedIn. https://www.linkedin.com/pulse/impact-culture-consistency-vs-motivation-farhad-heidari-phd-mba-gfgee
8. AMA. https://www.ama-assn.org/practice-management/scope-practice/physician-led-team-based-care
9. National Library of Medicine. https://www.ncbi.nlm.nih.gov/pmc/articles/PMC6361117/
10. AHRQ. https://www.ahrq.gov/patient-safety/patients-families/engagingfamilies/index.html
11. ISixSigma. https://www.isixsigma.com/sipoc-copis/sipoc-diagram/
12. American Society for Quality. https://asq.org/quality-resources/six-sigma
13. Cohen F. Dahl O. "Lean Six Sigma for the Medical Practice." Greenbranch Publishing, 2010.
14. Environmental Protection Agency. https://www.epa.gov/sustainability/lean-thinking-and-methods-5s

15. Miro. https://miro.com/blog/spaghetti-diagram/
16. Lean.org. https://www.lean.org/lexicon-terms/5-whys/
17. Virginia Mason Institute. https://www.virginiamasoninstitute.org/waste-walk/
18. U.S. Centers for Medicare and Medicaid Services. https://qpp.cms.gov/mips/traditional-mips
19. NLM. https://pubmed.ncbi.nlm.nih.gov/10114534/

Chapter 2

Administrative Structures in Medical Practice Operations

By: Dawn Plested, FACHE, MBA, JD, ESQ

"Efficiency is doing things right; effectiveness is doing the right things."

—Peter Drucker

2.1 Introduction

Administrative structures serve as the backbone of a medical practice, providing a foundation for all its operations. While medical schools teach expertise in providing clinical care, they often lack extensive training for healthcare providers on how to manage the administrative aspects of running a medical practice. Consequently, many physicians, despite their clinical excellence, may lack the knowledge and skills required to establish effective administrative structures when starting their practices.

Medical practices are complex organizations that require effective administrative structures beyond the provider themselves to ensure their efficient operation and compliance with regulations. This chapter will explore the significance of administrative structures and their role in advanced strategy and operations within a medical practice.

Importance of Administrative Structures

Effective administrative structures set the stage for medical practices to thrive and fulfill their mission of providing high-quality patient care. According to the American Medical Association, administrative structures are crucial to help promote methodical and flexible day-to-day operations with a patient-centered focus.[1] A robust and well-developed administrative structure offers many benefits to a medical practice or healthcare organization.

Well-designed structures and systems contribute to efficient operations and the smooth functioning of a practice, reducing operational bottlenecks and improving productivity. The efficient flow of patients and resources is essential for providing timely and high-quality care. Playing a pivotal role in the delivery of patient care, these structures help streamline processes, reduce errors and enhance the overall patient experience. From appointment scheduling to follow-up care, well-organized administrative processes ensure that patients receive consistent, reliable and coordinated care.

Aligning financial with clinical goals can be a challenge for medical practices. Reducing costs and improving financial status takes internal accountability. Administrative structures are vital for managing the practice's finances, ensuring that revenue flows smoothly while expenses are managed effectively. By adopting innovative financial strategies, administrative structures can skillfully balance budgets while prioritizing investments in technology and personnel. Comprehensive revenue management is essential for sustaining the practice and investing in further improvements. It's crucial to ensure that each financial decision positively impacts patient care by improving quality and maintaining accessibility.

Administrative structures also play a crucial role in compliance with healthcare regulations to avoid legal issues and penalties. Data privacy, clinical guidelines and labor laws are just some examples of the kinds of aspects that need internal monitoring from administrations. Maintaining a dedicated compliance team and partnering with compliance experts can help medical practices stay updated and adapt to evolving regulations. Administrative structures ensure that the practice adheres to these regulatory compliance issues, protecting both patients and the practice from potential legal ramifications and breaches of privacy.

Healthcare is an ever-changing environment and effective administrative structures enable practices to adapt to unforeseen challenges, such as the impact of events like the COVID-19 pandemic. Administrative adaptability and flexibility allows practices to pivot, accommodate new regulations and address emerging patient needs efficiently.

2.2 Leadership's Influence on Administrative Structures

"The best leaders are those most interested in surrounding themselves with assistants and associates smarter than they are."
—John C. Maxwell

Leadership is at the core of defining a practice's culture, which in turn, impacts its administrative structures. Different leadership models such as servant leadership, authoritative leadership or transformational leadership can influence decision-making, communication, patient and employee engagement, and patient satisfaction. The choice of leadership style has a profound impact on the practice's ability to pivot and adapt to changing circumstances.

Successful Leadership Approach to Administrative Structures

Effective leadership is not only about setting a vision but also about supporting and enabling the administrative structure that sustains and advances the practice's mission. According to Robert K. Greenleaf, author of *The Servant as Leader*, applying a successful leadership approach to administrative structures involves developing a methodology that recognizes and helps staff continually become better at their jobs.[2] That leadership approach should include several elements to ensure continuous organizational improvement.

Trusting and delegating responsibilities to staff is crucial for effective leadership. This allows the practice to function smoothly and staff can take ownership of their roles. Effective leaders empower their teams to make decisions and take initiative within their areas of responsibility. Leadership also defines the practice's culture. As a result, the culture should align with the practice's mission and values, fostering a patient-centered and purpose-driven work environment. Leaders who emphasize a culture of empathy, compassion and respect create a positive environment that benefits both patients and staff.

Providing growth opportunities for staff development and career advancement within the organization is another crucial element. A satisfied and motivated workforce is more likely to contribute positively to the practice's success. Leaders who invest in staff development, whether through training, mentorship, or educational opportunities, demonstrate a commitment to the long-term growth of their team. Foster a positive work environment where employees enjoy working together. A strong, collaborative team can significantly impact patient care and satisfaction. When employees experience a sense of belonging, they are more likely to deliver exceptional care and form strong relationships with patients.

Leadership that focuses on enhancing the experience of its employees through shared responsibilities and a formal range of training and personal enhancement programs can help drive a more successful practice with reduced employee turnover.

2.3 Organizational Design and Structure

Administrative structures in medical practices encompass a wide array of roles and functions that manage the non-clinical aspects of healthcare delivery. These structures encompass various administrative departments, each with a specific focus and purpose. They often include leadership roles like practice administrators, office managers and department heads who oversee various aspects of the practice's operations. Effective leadership sets the tone for the entire practice and plays a crucial role in decision-making, resource allocation and overall strategy.

Understanding the components and workflow of administrative structures is essential for ensuring the smooth operation of a medical practice, and, at the same time, helping to free up time for providers to offer more direct patient care. According to the AMA's Tanya Albert

Henry, nearly one-third of U.S. physicians spend more than 20 hours a week on paperwork and administrative tasks.[3] Consider the widely varied administrative roles performed throughout a healthcare practice and how they can work together to lighten that burden.

Front Office, Finance and Billing

The front office staff typically includes receptionists, appointment schedulers, and medical billing and coding specialists who handle patient interactions, appointments and billing. These frontline staff members are often the first point of contact for patients, making their roles critical for creating a positive patient experience. The finance and billing department manages financial matters, including insurance billing, accounts receivable, financial reporting and budgeting. As previously discussed, effective financial management is vital for ensuring the practice's financial sustainability and growth.

Human Resources and Compliance

Human Resources personnel are responsible for staff recruitment, training, payroll, benefits administration and employee relations. They play a crucial role in attracting and retaining qualified staff and promoting a positive workplace culture. The compliance and regulatory affairs team ensures that the practice complies with healthcare regulations, privacy laws (e.g., HIPAA), and accreditation requirements. Their work is essential for avoiding legal issues and ensuring the protection of patient data.

IT, QA and Performance Improvement

Information technology (IT) staff handle the practice's technology needs, including electronic health records (EHR) systems, practice management software and data security. Technology is an integral part of modern healthcare and IT departments are responsible for ensuring data accuracy, security, and accessibility. The quality assurance and performance improvement department focuses on maintaining and enhancing the quality of care and services provided by the practice. They monitor clinical and operational processes, identify areas for improvement and implement quality improvement initiatives.

Marketing and PR

Marketing and public relations professionals work on promoting the practice, managing its online presence and handling patient communications. Effective marketing and public relations can help attract new patients and build a strong practice brand. According to NIH, there are several benefits for healthcare organizations to implement marketing and PR strategies:[4]

- Improve the competitive advantage
- Increase the practice's visibility
- Create a solid reputation among patients and the community
- To understand the needs and expectations of consumers

Effective marketing and PR strategies ultimately help practices understand the patients' perceptions of the quality and results of their experience. This knowledge allows practices to offer memorable positive experiences to patients while building a strong, effective and dominant brand in the health services market.

Operations and Risk Management

Operations and facilities oversee the physical infrastructure, maintenance and the overall operational efficiency of the practice. The physical environment, equipment and facilities should be conducive to providing high-quality care. Risk management involves identifying and mitigating risks to the practice, such as legal, financial and safety-related risks. Effective risk management protects the practice and its patients from potential harm and legal consequences.

The specific administrative structure can vary depending on the size and complexity of the medical practice. Smaller practices may have fewer administrative roles, while larger practices or medical groups may have more elaborate structures. The ultimate goal of these administrative structures is to support healthcare professionals in providing quality care to patients while ensuring the practice runs efficiently, complies with regulations and maintains financial sustainability.

2.4 Choosing the Right Organizational Structure

"Organizational structure is the framework that helps employees achieve company goals. By defining employee roles and structure, it provides guidance on how to organize and manage company operations."

—The Balance Small Business

Selecting the appropriate organizational structure is a pivotal decision when establishing a medical practice. The choice should align with the practice's goals, size, patient population, specialization and regulatory considerations. The main types of organizational structures include solo practices, group practices, partnerships, hospital-owned practices and integrated health systems. According to the U.S. Small Business Administration, it's important to consider six factors when making a decision on the right kind of structure:[5]

- Goals and mission
- Level of autonomy and responsibility
- Size of practice
- Specialization
- Regulations
- Interoperability

Define your practice's goals and mission and determine what you aim to achieve in terms of patient care, community impact and financial sustainability. Your organizational structure should align with these goals. Determine the level of autonomy and responsibility you want in managing the practice. Solo practices offer complete autonomy while hospital-owned practices may involve less autonomy but more support in terms of resources and administrative services. Also consider the size of the practice and the patient population you aim to serve. Smaller practices may have a more straightforward organizational structure, while larger practices may involve more complex decision-making processes.

Assess the specialization of your practice and how it aligns with the chosen structure. Specialized practices may benefit from partnerships with other specialists or institutions that can complement their services.

Be aware of local, state and federal regulations relevant to your practice. Certain organizational structures may have specific regulatory requirements and compliance is essential to avoid legal issues. Finally, ensure that the organizational structure can adapt to new technologies and interoperability requirements. In the modern healthcare landscape, the ability to integrate with EHRs and other healthcare systems is crucial for sustainable success.

Selecting the right structure should be a thoughtful and strategic decision that reflects your practice's unique needs and long-term objectives.

2.5 Implementing Health Information Systems

> *"The adoption of health information technology, including electronic health records (EHRs), has the potential to provide substantial benefits to physicians, clinic practices, and health systems."*
> —American Medical Association (AMA)

Health information systems, such as EHRs and Practice Management Systems (PMS), are essential tools for medical practices. These systems help automate processes, improve efficiency, and enhance patient care. The AMA's "Digital Health Implementation Playbook" recommends a measured approach when implementing health information systems.[6]

Identify Needs and Customize Technology

Start with identifying your practice's specific needs and requirements before choosing and implementing any health information system. A one-size-fits-all approach may not be suitable for all practices. Customize your technology solutions to meet the unique demands of your patients and clinical workflows. Ensure that your EHR and practice management systems can seamlessly integrate with other tools and technologies. Interoperability is crucial for efficient data exchange and collaboration with other healthcare providers. In a patient's healthcare journey, information must flow seamlessly between primary care, specialists, labs and hospitals.

Choose systems that offer a user-friendly design to reduce the learning curve for staff and healthcare providers. User-friendly interfaces improve staff satisfaction and can reduce the risk of user errors. A well-designed user interface contributes to better user adoption and system efficiency. Invest in training for your staff and create standardized processes to ensure consistent use of the system. Standardized processes minimize errors, improve data accuracy and facilitate better communication between healthcare providers and support staff.

Emphasize Adaptability and Continuous Improvement

Stay informed about emerging technologies and their potential to enhance your practice's efficiency; adaptability and flexibility are critical. Technology in healthcare evolves rapidly, so it's important to adapt to new tools and strategies. Keeping an eye on industry trends and innovations can give your practice a competitive edge. Emphasize continuous quality improvement to optimize processes, reduce errors and enhance patient care. Continuous quality improvement involves regularly assessing your administrative and clinical processes and making incremental changes to improve efficiency and effectiveness. Establish a mechanism for regular reporting and analysis of your system's performance. This includes monitoring areas like Accounts Receivable (AR), billing, denials, expenses and revenues. Regular reporting helps identify potential issues and provides data-driven insights for making improvements.

By effectively implementing and utilizing health information systems, you can improve the overall efficiency and quality of care within your practice. Health information systems help reduce administrative burden, enhance patient engagement and ensure that healthcare providers have access to critical patient data at the point of care.

2.6 Financial Management

Financial management is a critical component of operating a successful medical practice. This aspect encompasses various tasks including budgeting, financial planning, revenue cycle management (RCM) and implementing strategies for cost optimization and revenue enhancement. Proper financial management ensures that the practice remains financially sustainable while providing high-quality patient care.

Budgeting and Financial Planning

Budgeting and financial planning are essential for maintaining the financial health of a medical practice. These processes involve creating a comprehensive financial plan that outlines expected revenues, expenses and financial goals. Key considerations include:

- **Revenue projections:** Accurately estimate the practice's revenue based on patient volume, services offered and payor mix.
- **Expense budget:** Plan for operational expenses, including staff salaries, rent, utilities and supplies.
- **Capital expenditure:** Allocate funds for necessary equipment, technology and facility improvements.
- **Emergency fund:** Set aside reserves for unexpected expenses or economic downturns.
- **Investment strategy:** Determine how surplus funds will be invested to generate returns.

By establishing a well-structured budget and financial plan, a medical practice can proactively manage its finances and make informed decisions regarding investments and cost control.

Revenue Cycle Management (RCM)

According to the American Academy of Professional Coders (AAPC), the revenue cycle encompasses the entire patient journey, from appointment scheduling to billing and collections.[7] Effectively managing this one aspect is vital for optimizing revenue and maintaining financial stability. Key RCM components include:

- **Appointment scheduling:** Efficient scheduling minimizes patient wait times, reduces idle staff hours, and optimizes provider productivity.
- **Insurance verification:** Accurate verification of patient insurance details helps prevent claim denials and delayed payments.
- **Patient registration:** Ensure that patient information is collected accurately to prevent billing errors.
- **Coding and documentation:** Accurate medical coding and comprehensive documentation are crucial for successful claims submission.

Chapter 2: Administrative Structures in Medical Practice Operations

- **Claims submission and management:** Streamline the process of submitting claims to insurance providers and actively manage the claims process to minimize denials.
- **Billing and collections:** Timely billing and effective collections procedures are essential for maintaining a healthy cash flow.

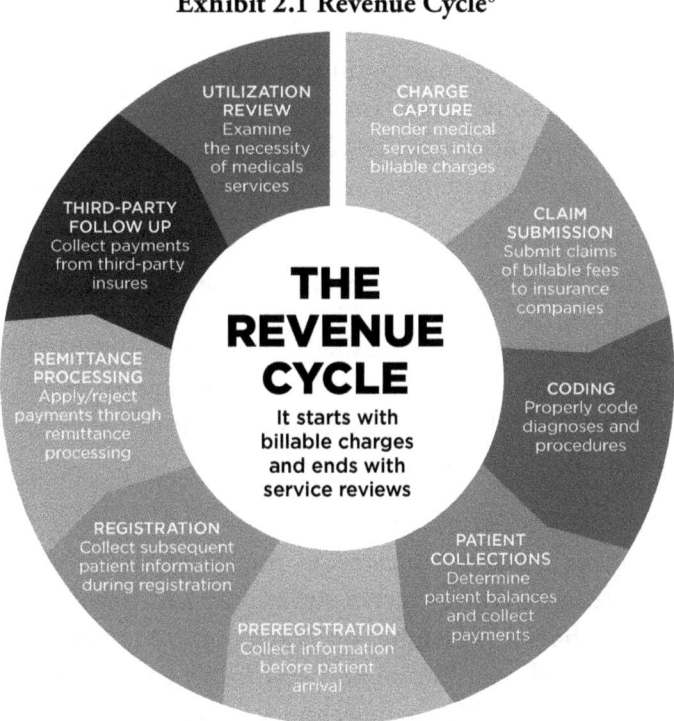

Exhibit 2.1 Revenue Cycle[8]

THE REVENUE CYCLE — It starts with billable charges and ends with service reviews

- **UTILIZATION REVIEW:** Examine the necessity of medicals services
- **CHARGE CAPTURE:** Render medical services into billable charges
- **CLAIM SUBMISSION:** Submit claims of billable fees to insurance companies
- **CODING:** Properly code diagnoses and procedures
- **PATIENT COLLECTIONS:** Determine patient balances and collect payments
- **PREREGISTRATION:** Collect information before patient arrival
- **REGISTRATION:** Collect subsequent patient information during registration
- **REMITTANCE PROCESSING:** Apply/reject payments through remittance processing
- **THIRD-PARTY FOLLOW UP:** Collect payments from third-party insures

Accounts Receivable Management

Tracking your accounts receivable monthly allows providers to identify those at risk of becoming leaked revenue and contributing to bad debt. ARs can then be compared over time to recognize dangerous trends early and determine any outstanding reimbursements that may prove easy to close. According to PayrHealth, providers should analyze their AR data to determine aged debtors and collection rates—two metrics that provide an overview of providers' AR cycles.[9] Aged debtor reports reveal how many receivable accounts exist within each age group, while collection rates demonstrate how successful providers are at converting ARs to reimbursements in a given accounting period.

When tracking AR, determine if there is a delay between providing care and invoicing. Longer ARs can become forgotten by patients, leading to unpaid invoices. By starting the cycle as early as possible, providers can keep them from aging beyond collection. From there, determine how long the different stages of the cycle take to identify opportunities for improvements..

Monitor and manage outstanding accounts receivable to ensure that payments are received promptly. Implementing technology such as EHRs and practice management systems (PMS) can significantly enhance RCM by automating various processes, reducing errors and improving billing efficiency.

Strategies for Cost Optimization and Revenue Enhancement

Medical practices are increasingly turning to advanced strategies to optimize costs and enhance revenue. Lamont Louis, MBA, CEO of Einstein Physicians Philadelphia, suggests the value of a proactive strategy, which includes many of the following tools:[10]

- **Telemedicine services:** The adoption of telemedicine allows practices to expand their services, reach a broader patient base, and reduce overhead costs associated with in-person visits.
- **Value-based care models:** Transitioning to value-based care models can lead to cost savings by emphasizing preventive care, reducing unnecessary tests and treatments and improving patient outcomes.
- **Population health management:** Implement population health management programs to identify at-risk patient populations and proactively address their healthcare needs, reducing the cost of treating chronic illnesses.
- **Partnerships and collaborations:** Collaborate with other healthcare providers or institutions to share resources, reduce costs and access specialized services.
- **Data analytics:** Utilize data analytics to identify trends, patterns and opportunities for cost reduction or revenue

enhancement. Data-driven decisions are becoming increasingly important in healthcare management.

- **Patient-centered medical homes (PCMH):** Transform the practice into a PCMH, emphasizing patient-centered care, care coordination and access to various healthcare services within the medical home.

Incorporating robust financial management practices into the administrative structure of a medical practice ensures that it remains fiscally responsible, efficient and capable of delivering exceptional patient care. The interplay between budgeting, RCM and advanced financial strategies is integral to achieving long-term financial success. These advanced strategies focus on providing high-quality care while optimizing costs, which is essential for the financial sustainability of the practice. *Vol. 1: Advanced Strategy for Medical Practice Leaders: Financial Management Edition* provides clear and in depth financial management strategies that can be incorporated into any healthcare organization.

2.7 Enhancing Patient Engagement and Satisfaction

"The quality of the patient experience is tied directly to the degree of their engagement in their care."
—American Academy of Family Physicians (AAFP)

Successful medical practices share the same essential element: patient engagement and satisfaction. A patient-centric approach in the administrative process can significantly impact how patients perceive and interact with your practice. The American College of Physicians' "Patients Before Paperwork" initiative is one example of a concerted effort to reduce the administrative burden and heighten the focus on patients.[11] To help better engage patients, consider the following key steps:

1. **Open communication:** Establish a two-way communication process that allows patients to feel heard and valued. Address their questions, concerns and feedback promptly. Open communication fosters trust and ensures that patients are actively involved in their care.

2. **Streamline patient touchpoints:** Identify areas in the patient journey, such as scheduling, in-office experience and results follow-up, where you can streamline processes to improve patient satisfaction. Reducing wait times, enhancing appointment scheduling and providing convenient access to test results are all areas where administrative improvements can lead to higher patient satisfaction.

3. **Open multiple communication channels:** Offer patients multiple communication channels—such as online scheduling, phone calls or text messages—to accommodate their preferences. Diverse communication options ensure that patients can engage with your practice in ways that are most convenient for them.

4. **Implement patient-centric design:** Design administrative processes with the patient in mind, focusing on what would enhance their experience and convenience. For example, optimizing your practice's website for easy navigation and online appointment scheduling can significantly enhance the patient experience. Patient-centric design extends to all touchpoints, including signage, patient portals and phone interactions.

5. **Emphasize continuous improvement:** Prioritize continuous quality improvement initiatives to maintain and enhance the patient-centered approach throughout your practice. Regularly seek patient feedback, conduct surveys, and implement improvements based on patient input. Patient feedback is a valuable source of information for identifying areas of improvement and addressing patient concerns.

Patient engagement and satisfaction should remain at the forefront of your practice's goals with a commitment to delivering high-quality and patient-centric care. The administrative team plays a critical role in creating an environment that fosters patient engagement and ensures a positive patient experience.

2.8 Navigating Legal and Regulatory Compliance

"Efforts to ensure compliance should always be viewed as a valuable investment in the organization's future, not just as an added cost."
—Foley & Lardner LLP

The medical field is subject to numerous laws and regulations that affect how practices operate. Administrative structures must facilitate adherence to these regulations to avoid legal issues. Stay informed about relevant laws, such as the Health Insurance Portability and Accountability Act (HIPAA), the Affordable Care Act (ACA) and state-specific regulations. The U.S. Department of Health and Human Services (HHS) publication, "HIPAA for Professionals," offers a comprehensive overview of compliance strategies, and suggests practices invest in the following measures to help meet compliance regulations:[12]

Training and Education

Ensure that all staff members receive training on relevant regulations. Educational programs and ongoing training are crucial to ensure that everyone in the practice understands their compliance responsibilities. Develop and maintain policies and procedures that reflect legal and regulatory requirements. Periodically review and update them to ensure they remain up-to-date and aligned with evolving regulations.

Data Security

Implement and maintain strong privacy and security measures, especially concerning patient data. Data breaches can lead to severe consequences, including financial penalties and damage to the practice's reputation. Robust data security measures and encryption are essential to protect sensitive patient information. HIPAA requires healthcare organizations to secure and protect patient information, so it is imperative to ensure your staff is trained and updated on HIPAA laws and best practices.

Continuous Monitoring

Conduct regular audits to ensure compliance and monitor practice activities that may impact compliance. Monitoring helps identify potential issues early and provides an opportunity to address them before they result in legal repercussions. When in doubt or facing complex legal situations, consult legal experts who specialize in healthcare law. Legal counsel can provide guidance on complex issues and help ensure that your practice complies with the law.

Compliance with healthcare regulations is a fundamental responsibility of medical practices. While administrative structures play a significant role in achieving compliance, it is a collective effort involving every member of the practice along with outside help. Join and stay active in professional associations to access resources and information related to legal and regulatory changes in healthcare. These associations often provide valuable updates on changing regulations and best practices for compliance. Maintain comprehensive records of compliance efforts, including training records, audit results, and communication with legal experts. Proper documentation demonstrates the practice's commitment to compliance, which can be valuable in the event of a legal inquiry.

2.9 Measuring Administrative Efficiency and Performance

"To improve is to change; to be perfect is to change often."
—Winston Churchill

Efficiency and performance measurement is an ongoing process that helps practices identify areas for improvement and enhance overall operations. Resources such as the AMA's Practice Innovation Strategies suggest tracking workflows and using analytics to help gauge the success of administrative systems, and make process changes wherever necessary.[13] There are several measurement tools that can help assess administrative efficiency and performance.

KPIs and Benchmarking

Identify and track key performance indicators (KPIs) that measure different aspects of administrative performance. KPIs may include patient wait times, appointment scheduling accuracy, billing accuracy and revenue collections. Regularly assess these metrics to identify trends and areas for improvement. Compare your practice's administrative performance to industry benchmarks or best practices. Benchmarking can help identify areas where your practice excels and areas that require improvement. Leveraging the best practices of other successful practices can lead to meaningful changes and efficiency gains.

Feedback

Conduct patient satisfaction surveys to collect feedback and insights into administrative performance. Patient feedback is invaluable in understanding their experience with your practice. Identify areas where patients express dissatisfaction and take corrective action. Also assess how effectively your practice utilizes technology to streamline administrative processes. Evaluate the performance and ROI of your health information systems, appointment scheduling tools, and practice management software. Ensure that technology is optimized to support the practice's goals.

Lean Six Sigma

Encourage a culture of continuous process improvement within your practice. Staff should feel empowered to suggest changes that enhance efficiency and patient satisfaction. As discussed in the previous chapter, consider implementing Lean or Six Sigma methodologies to systematically identify and address inefficiencies. Review how time and resources are allocated within your practice. Ensure that staff are spending their time on tasks that align with the practice's goals. Reallocation of resources to high-impact areas can significantly improve efficiency. Effectively manage changes within your administrative structures. Any significant changes, such as adopting a new EHR system or restructuring the front office, should be carefully planned and executed. A structured approach to change management can mitigate potential disruptions and resistance from staff.

Measuring administrative efficiency and performance is an ongoing effort that should involve the entire administrative team. Regular assessments, feedback loops and strategic adjustments contribute to a practice that operates at its highest potential.

2.10 Practice in Action

Boston Children's Hospital initiated a program which employed advanced technology to optimize its administrative processes.[14] While the hospital is world-renowned for its innovative robotic surgery research and training program, which uses minimally invasive surgery procedures and shares those with other institutions, it suffered from the old-fashioned burden of paper records.

A range of workflow automation tools were implemented with the ultimate goal of improving patient care, by lessening the burden of administrative staff and providing patients with more technology-based options for both direct and remote care.

The hospital, a 347-bed pediatric center with 18,000 inpatient admissions and more than 300,000 emergency care patients per year, is one of the largest pediatric medical facilities in the country. The hospital still relied on paper-based patient records, many stretching back to the 1960s, taking up valuable physical space and consuming staff time to access and transfer between departments.

A first effort was the full replacement of paper records with a suite of digital documents using a single, hospital-wide system, resulting in more than $2 million a year in cost savings. This system integrated existing workflows but enhanced options for inter-departmental collaboration, as well as the secure transfer of documentation.

The hospital also adopted a variety of digitized tools to help with other administrative processes. Robotics process automation (RPA) is now used to help automate repetitive tasks in coding and document processing. RPA technology has been used to automate labor-intensive, multistep tasks, freeing up administrative staff to other tasks. The state health authority, MassHealth, has established a full RPA policy, which requires approval to use automation and robotics on Medicaid management systems and the Provider Online Service Center.[15]

As many healthcare organizations did during the pandemic, the hospital has also moved to digital health tools including telehealth platforms, which allow more remote patient consultations.

2.11 Summary

Administrative structures are the foundation upon which successful medical practices are built. This chapter explored the vital role of

Chapter 2: Administrative Structures in Medical Practice Operations

administrative structures in healthcare operations. Effective administrative structures contribute to efficient practice operations, regulatory compliance, patient-centered care, and financial sustainability.

- Leadership within a medical practice plays a critical role in defining its culture and approach to administrative structures. Leadership styles and approaches significantly influence decision-making, staff engagement and patient satisfaction.
- Selecting the right organizational structure is a strategic decision that should align with the practice's goals, size, specialization and regulatory considerations. The choice of structure can have profound implications for the practice's autonomy, responsibility and future direction.
- Health information systems are fundamental tools for modern medical practices. Implementing these systems effectively can reduce administrative burden, streamline workflows and enhance patient care.
- Patient engagement and satisfaction are essential components of a successful practice. Focusing on open communication, streamlined patient touchpoints and continuous quality improvement can lead to a positive patient experience.
- Compliance with legal and regulatory requirements is a fundamental responsibility for medical practices. Establishing educational programs, policies and procedures, and a culture of compliance is crucial for avoiding legal issues.
- Measuring administrative efficiency and performance involves tracking key performance indicators, benchmarking, patient surveys, technology utilization and process improvement initiatives. A structured approach to performance assessment supports ongoing improvements in practice operations.
- Effective administrative structures are an essential part of a thriving medical practice, enabling it to fulfill its mission of providing high-quality, patient-centered care.

In summary, the administrative structures of a medical practice play a multifaceted and crucial role in its success. By addressing each of the topics covered in this chapter, practices can develop a comprehensive understanding of how administrative structures impact various aspects of healthcare operations and implement strategies to ensure that any practice operates efficiently and effectively.

In the next chapter, we will look at staffing and operations management in the healthcare setting, including a variety of financial and operational staffing indicators and models. We will also discuss recruitment, retention, outsourcing and focus on labor laws applicable for operational leaders, as well as provide details on integrating the notions of Diversity, Equity and Inclusion (DEI) into staffing and operations oversight.

Notes

1. AMA. https://www.ama-assn.org/practice-management/reducing-administrative-burden
2. Center for Servant Leadership. https://www.greenleaf.org/what-is-servant-leadership/
3. AMA. https://www.ama-assn.org/practice-management/sustainability/do-you-spend-more-time-administrative-tasks-your-peers
4. NIH. https://www.ncbi.nlm.nih.gov/pmc/articles/PMC6685306/
5. SBA. https://www.sba.gov/business-guide/launch-your-business/choose-business-structure
6. AMA. https://www.ama-assn.org/practice-management/digital/digital-health-implementation-playbook-series
7. AAPC. https://www.aapc.com/resources/what-is-revenue-cycle-management
8. Tech Target. https://www.techtarget.com/searchhealthit/definition/revenue-cycle-management-RCM
9. PayrHealth. https://payrhealth.com/blog/how-to-improve-your-accounts-receivable-ar-in-healthcare
10. MGMA. https://www.mgma.com/articles/from-reactive-to-proactive-essential-medical-practice-financial-metrics-and-key-performance-indicators
11. ACP. https://www.acponline.org/advocacy/where-we-stand/patients-before-paperwork-reducing-administrative-burdens
12. HHS. https://www.hhs.gov/hipaa/for-professionals/index.html
13. AMA. https://www.ama-assn.org/practice-management/ama-steps-forward/practice-innovation-strategies-time-saving-strategies
14. Tungsten Automation. https://www.tungstenautomation.com/learn/case-studies/2019/cs_boston-childrens-hospital_en
15. Mass.gov. https://www.mass.gov/guides/masshealth-robotics-processing-automation-rpa-policy

Chapter 3

Staffing and Operations

By: Adrienne Palmer Lloyd,
MHA, FACHE

3.1 Introduction

One constant remains throughout healthcare: the pivotal role of a proficient and highly-skilled workforce that is seamlessly aligned with leadership to create an exceptional patient environment and drive outstanding results.

The quality of care provided, the attainment of an organization's mission and vision, and the realization of goals all hinge on the strength of the healthcare workforce. Healthcare leaders' capacity to unlock the full potential of their teams is key to any organization's success.

This chapter delves into the intricate world of healthcare workforce management, with a specific focus on operations and staffing. We will cover the essential components that contribute to creating a high-functioning healthcare team—one that is not only well-prepared to meet the demands of modern healthcare but also aligned with the core values and objectives of your organization.

Here is a brief overview of what to expect as we explore the various components of operations and staffing necessary to build a team that works with you and your organization to drive success:

- Financial and Operational Staffing Indicators
- Staffing Models
- Recruitment and Retention
- Outsourcing and Automation
- Diversity, Equity and Inclusion (DEI)
- Labor Laws for Operational Leaders

Leadership can be especially challenging in healthcare, but understanding the key areas and taking steps to designing a team that works with you and is aligned with your organization's goals can drive great results.

3.2 Key Financial and Operational Staffing Indicators

Navigating Staffing Efficiency and Effectiveness

In healthcare, the management of staffing is a critical aspect that significantly impacts both financial stability and operational effectiveness. According to Amwins, a medical insurance provider, staffing plays a vital role in maintaining the quality of care provided to patients, and ensuring that they receive the attention and expertise that they need.[1] Understanding and effectively managing key financial and operational staffing indicators is essential for healthcare leaders aiming to optimize their workforce while maintaining high standards of patient care.

Financial Indicators Related to Staffing

- **Staffing Expense Ratio:** This indicator measures staffing costs as a percentage of total revenue. It's crucial for understanding the proportion of revenue consumed by staffing expenses. A higher ratio may indicate overstaffing or high labor costs, while a lower ratio could suggest understaffing or efficient labor management.
- **Labor Cost per Patient Day:** This measures the average cost of labor for each day a patient spends in the facility. It helps in assessing how labor costs are tracking against patient care activities.

- **Overtime Percentage:** Monitoring the percentage of total labor hours that are overtime can indicate staffing inefficiencies, potential burnout or inadequate staffing levels.
- **Benefit Cost as a Percentage of Total Salary:** This ratio highlights the cost of employee benefits relative to total salaries. It's essential for understanding the full cost of staffing beyond just salaries. According to the International Foundation of Employee Benefit Plans, benefits costs continue to average approximately 30% of payroll costs.[2]

Operational Staffing Indicators

- **Staff Turnover Rate:** High turnover rates can be costly and disrupt patient care continuity. Monitoring this helps in understanding employee satisfaction and retention effectiveness.
- **Staff-to-Patient Ratio:** This ratio is vital for ensuring adequate staffing levels to meet patient care needs without overstaffing. Appropriate staffing levels are crucial for both quality care and operational efficiency.
- **Time-to-Fill Vacancies:** Measures the average time taken to fill open positions. Longer times can indicate challenges in attracting talent or inefficiencies in the recruitment process.
- **Employee Productivity Metrics:** These metrics, such as patients seen per provider per day or clinical procedures performed per staff member, help in assessing how effectively staff time is utilized.[3] These can include FTE per work relative value unit (wRVU), case, procedure or visits.[4] Additionally, you will want to consider how overtime plays into the FTE total and overall costs as compared to your patient demands.
- **Provider Productivity Metrics:** Measures the efficiency and effectiveness of providers, including patient volume, service variety, and outcomes.

Utilizing Staffing Indicators for Strategic Management

To make the most of these staffing indicators, healthcare leaders should take a number of steps to put them into action. Most importantly, they should regularly monitor and analyze these indicators to help identify trends, issues and other areas for improvement. Benchmarking, using industry standards such as the MGMA DataDive Operations Metrics, can be helpful in gauging staffing metrics.[5] Benchmarking can identify best practices and design improvement initiatives to increase performance and efficiency where possible—through technology integration, additional staff training, process changes or staffing model shifts.

Managers should also use these metrics to develop strategic staffing plans to inform staffing strategies, ensuring alignment with patient care demands and financial constraints. Investments in staff development will help ensure that staff are well-trained and equipped to provide efficient and high-quality care. Better integration of technology can also be beneficial in streamlining staffing processes, from scheduling to performance monitoring. There should also be an ongoing focus on employee engagement. According to the CDC, engagement results in improved employee and customer satisfaction, safety and overall performance and profits.[6] Engaged staff are more productive and contribute to a positive work environment, impacting both operational and financial outcomes.

Future Trends: Predictive Analytics in Staffing

The next frontier in staffing is the use of predictive analytics. By leveraging historical data, healthcare leaders can forecast staffing needs and preemptively adjust schedules and staff levels to optimize both operations and budget.[7] There are software products and technologies that have been helping with this to a small degree on the inpatient staffing side, but these are beginning to be more prevalent in the outpatient setting as well and this will only continue to expand with the implementation of artificial intelligence (AI) into these solutions.

Effective management of staffing in healthcare is a delicate balance of ensuring sufficient, skilled and engaged personnel while maintaining financial prudence. It can also produce profound results for patients.

States with staffing mandates have shown fewer surgery-related deaths, less time spent in the ICU and increased patient satisfaction.[8] By closely monitoring and strategically responding to key financial and operational staffing indicators, healthcare leaders can optimize their workforce, enhance patient care and achieve organizational goals. These indicators are not just metrics; they are the pulse of the organization, signaling the health of staffing practices and their impact on the broader healthcare ecosystem.

3.3 Optimizing Staffing Models in Healthcare

Effective staffing models are essential for delivering high-quality healthcare services while managing costs. As a healthcare leader, you must carefully design staffing models that strike a balance between patient care and operational efficiency. Staffing is a critical aspect of medical practice operations, and the challenges involved in recruiting and retaining qualified personnel have become more pronounced in recent years. According to the Association of American Colleges, the United States could see an estimated shortage of between 37,800 and 124,000 physicians by 2034.[9] Other medical support roles have been equally impacted by changing labor markets, since the pandemic. To ensure efficient operations, consider the following when staffing your organization.

- **Cost management:** Staffing is often one of the largest costs for a medical practice. Allocate resources to cover staffing needs and ensure that your budget aligns with your staffing plans. Effective cost management helps maintain financial sustainability and ensures that resources are allocated where they are most needed.
- **Recruitment and retention:** Develop effective recruitment and retention strategies to attract and keep qualified staff. Competitive compensation packages, benefits and opportunities for career growth are essential for staff retention. Healthcare professionals are in high demand and offering attractive employment packages is vital for attracting and retaining talent.

- **Training:** Invest in training and standardize your training processes. Ensure that employees are well-trained and have clear expectations for their roles. Proper training enhances staff competence and helps them perform their duties with confidence and accuracy.
- **Cultural fit:** Create a workplace culture that values purpose-driven work, employee engagement and positive work environments. A satisfied and motivated workforce can have a significant impact on patient care. Cultivating a positive and inclusive culture can reduce staff turnover and improve the overall work environment.
- **Flexibility and adaptability:** Be prepared to adapt to changing staffing needs, especially in times of labor shortages and increased burnout rates within the healthcare industry. Staffing needs can fluctuate, and practices should have contingency plans and strategies to address staff shortages or surpluses.

Strategic staffing is an ongoing process that should align with your practice's goals and patient care requirements. By investing in the right people and creating a positive work environment, your practice can operate more efficiently and provide high-quality care.

Types of Staffing Models

Strategies in staffing models continue to evolve from the once-prevalent ideas of predetermined numbers to more flexible and technologically-enhanced models. The advent of collaborative care and the notions of outsourcing are also important in staffing plans that reflect contemporary healthcare realities. Consider the following staffing models along with their benefits and drawbacks:

Traditional Staffing Models: Traditional models in healthcare revolve around fixed staffing ratios, often mandated by regulatory bodies or institutional policies. This model relies heavily on a predetermined nurse-to-patient ratio or similar benchmarks for other healthcare professionals. While providing a straightforward approach, this model often lacks the flexibility to adapt to fluctuating patient needs and can lead to either understaffing or overstaffing.

Chapter 3: Staffing and Operations

Flexible Staffing Models: Flexible models, such as the use of float pools or per diem staff, allow healthcare facilities to adjust staffing levels based on real-time demand. This approach can improve efficiency and reduce costs associated with overtime or underutilization of staff. However, it requires effective communication and a strong understanding of the varying skill sets within the team. At Chicago's Rush University Medical Center, an ongoing staffing-to-demand (S2D) study has been used to calculate cycle times and help better meet patient demands through more flexible staffing planning.[10]

Team-Based Models: Team-based models focus on collaborative care, often involving multidisciplinary teams working together to provide comprehensive patient care. This model promotes better patient outcomes and staff satisfaction but requires strong leadership to coordinate and manage the diverse skills and roles within the team.

Technology-Enhanced Models: Emerging models integrate technology, like telemedicine and AI-assisted diagnostics, to extend the reach and effectiveness of healthcare staff. These models can enhance service delivery, especially in remote or underserved areas, but require significant investment in technology and training. According to ShiftMed, 35% of healthcare organizations surveyed have already implemented AI to assist with repetitive administrative tasks.[11]

Outsourcing vs In-house Models: With the onset of increased remote work and, most recently, AI technology, there are a growing number of options for leaders to consider as they consider approaches that will provide the best service for their patients while optimizing efficiency and margins. Options fall into two buckets: outsourcing through a company that provides staffing services and companies offering technologically enhanced solutions. These groups can either take over an entire process for your organization, a portion of one or offer solutions that will make it easier and more effective for you and your team to perform at your best.

Here is a table outlining various outsourcing options in healthcare, detailing areas where staffing agencies are commonly used alongside opportunities for technology solutions:

Exhibit 3.1 Outsourcing Options in Healthcare

Key Areas for Outsourcing through Staffing Agencies	Key Areas for Outsourcing or Enhancing through Technology Solutions
Revenue Cycle Management	Telemedicine for remote consultations
Patient Access/Scheduling	AI-assisted Triage Systems
Virtual Medical Assistants and Virtual Scribes	Automated Patient Scheduling and Reminders
Locum Physician, Nurse and Technologist Pools	Artificial Intelligence in Digital Imaging and Analysis
Patient Wellness and Group Coaching Programs	Wearable Health Technology that Provides Data to Providers
MIPS and PQI Monitoring and Care Coordination	Remote Patient Monitoring (RPM)

As with any change management, I recommend involving your team members in the analysis, vendor review, selection and implementation processes to ensure the changes are as smooth as possible and your current team understands the role of any supplemental solution.

Key Considerations When Selecting Staffing Models

Choosing the right staffing model is not a one-size-fits-all decision. It requires a thorough understanding of the specific needs of the healthcare facility, patient demographics and available resources. As a first step, consider metrics and process analysis. Key performance indicators (KPIs), such as patient satisfaction scores, staff turnover rates and financial metrics like cost-per-patient-day, are essential for evaluating staffing models.[12] Process analysis, often using Lean and Six Sigma methodologies, can identify inefficiencies and areas for improvement in existing staffing structures.

Technology can also be used as an evaluation tool. Healthcare leaders can leverage technology to gather real-time data on patient flow, staff utilization, and resource allocation. Advanced analytics and predictive modeling can forecast patient demand, helping leaders make informed decisions about staffing needs. As well, consider adopting a culture of continuous improvement and adaptation. According to the AMA, physicians often overlook the capabilities of administration staff and take on more responsibilities than necessary; by examining those processes and committing to ongoing improvements, additional staffing can help produce better outcomes and less stress for providers.[13] The healthcare landscape is continuously evolving, necessitating an adaptable approach to staffing. Regularly reviewing and adjusting the staffing model based on ongoing metrics and feedback is essential for maintaining optimal performance and patient care.

There are several key things to remember when you are evaluating which staffing models will be right for your team.

Patient-Centered Staffing

Ensure that your staffing models prioritize patient needs. This means considering factors like nurse-patient ratios, physician availability, and support staff to enhance patient satisfaction and safety. According to Karlene Kerfoot, CNO at API Healthcare, effective staffing is linked to patient safety, patient and workforce satisfaction, and operational outcomes in healthcare organizations.[14] Patient-centered staffing is not solely about numbers; it's about ensuring that the right staff with the right skills are available to provide timely and effective care. Leaders should collaborate with clinical teams to determine appropriate staffing levels based on patient acuity and workload and regularly seek feedback to adjust as needed.

Flexibility and Adaptability

Healthcare staffing models must be flexible to respond to fluctuations in patient volumes, seasonal demands and unexpected events like pandemics. Cross-training and resource sharing can be valuable strategies. Flexibility in staffing is crucial for responding to the dynamic nature of healthcare. Leaders should establish contingency plans for scenarios like surges in patient admissions or unexpected staff shortages. Cross-training employees in different roles and fostering a culture of adaptability can ensure that the organization can pivot effectively in challenging situations.

Technology Integration

Leverage technology to optimize staffing. Electronic health records (EHRs), telemedicine, and predictive analytics can assist in resource allocation and staff scheduling. Technology can enhance the efficiency of staffing models. EHR systems can provide real-time data on patient acuity and workload, allowing leaders to make informed staffing decisions. Telemedicine can extend the reach of healthcare providers, reducing the need for on-site staffing in some cases, but will also require active reskilling and cross-training to allow employees to provide more flexible and efficient use of telemedicine processes for patients.[15] Predictive analytics can help forecast patient volumes and staffing requirements, enabling proactive adjustments to staffing levels.

Skill Mix

Consider the skill mix within your healthcare team when designing staffing models. Optimal skill utilization can improve efficiency and enhance patient care. Leaders should assess the skill mix of their healthcare teams to ensure that the right professionals are available to address patient needs. For example, in an emergency department, having a mix of triage nurses, physician assistants and emergency physicians can optimize care delivery. Regularly evaluating skill utilization and aligning it with patient demand is essential.

The right staffing model in healthcare is dependent on a multitude of factors, including patient needs, staff skill sets and available resources. By utilizing a data-driven approach, incorporating technology and applying rigorous process analysis, healthcare leaders can effectively determine and implement the staffing model that best suits their specific situation—ultimately leading to enhanced patient care, staff satisfaction and organizational success.

3.4 Recruitment and Retention

Recruiting and retaining top talent in healthcare is an ongoing challenge, given the competitive nature of the industry and the importance of a skilled and motivated workforce. According to the American

Hospital Association, factors such as COVID-19 and the "great resignation" mean that the employment landscape has vastly changed, with employees seeking opportunities where they feel valued and rewarded for their work.[16]

Recruitment is the first step in building a high-performing healthcare team. Leaders should develop a recruitment strategy that aligns with the organization's mission and values. This includes identifying the qualities and skills sought in candidates and crafting compelling job postings. Building relationships with educational institutions can facilitate early access to emerging talent in healthcare.

Before posting the position, take the time to think through the following:

- What the role should be
- If any adjustments should be made
- Whether to replace the exact same role or consider looking at different staffing or outsourcing

Take each opening as an opportunity to assess the needs of the team and the organization. This does not need to be a lengthy process, but it is worth pausing and reflecting in line with what you are trying to create.

Recruitment Strategies

The aftermath of the pandemic helped healthcare organizations realize that employees have much different expectations and far more options available to them, making recruiting a far bigger challenge. Recruitment efforts now require more planning and the integration of various programs designed to sell your benefits as an employer, in order to attract and retain top talent.

Your organization's reputation and brand play a significant role in attracting top talent. Without a positive one, candidates may very well "swipe left" on you before they even read your posting. By ensuring your healthcare facility's reputation for committing to patient care, employee development and a positive work environment, you increase the chances of attracting high-performing candidates. According to KNB Communications, this requires tactics such as leveraging patient testimonials and closely monitoring your brand reputation by immediately addressing any negative comments or reviews left on your website.[17]

Today it is just as, if not more important, to manage your organization's online presence with social media and work engagement platforms such as LinkedIn, Google Reviews, Facebook, Indeed, etc. Many potential candidates will be reviewing your profile and feedback on these platforms more closely than they will follow your organization's website. It is critical to know what publicly exists and to take steps to ensure it portrays the image you want for your organization.

Take key steps like highlighting and celebrating not only your physicians' and other clinicians' academic or other achievements alongside patient stories, but also employee successes, work anniversaries or team building activities. This can help employees connect with your current team even before they apply and illustrate to them that you provide a culture highlight where they can feel seen and valued as individuals while contributing to the larger goals.

Implement a comprehensive talent acquisition strategy that includes attracting candidates through various channels. Job fairs, online platforms and professional networks are valuable sources for identifying potential employees. Consider establishing partnerships with educational institutions to nurture talent pipelines. According to Kimedics, other important acquisition strategies include streamlining the hiring process and prioritizing candidate experience to help seek out talented employees.[18]

Embrace and leverage technology in your recruitment efforts. Applicant tracking systems (ATS) can streamline the hiring process by managing applications, scheduling interviews and assessing candidate qualifications. Additionally, consider using video interviews to save time and resources during initial screening. Implement structured interview processes to ensure consistency and fairness in candidate assessments. Develop interview guides with standardized questions that evaluate

Chapter 3: Staffing and Operations

candidates' skills, experience and cultural fit. Include multiple stakeholders in the interview panel to gain diverse perspectives. Behavioral or situational interviewing can be very helpful to better understand how candidates approach situations, address challenges, lead initiatives, etc. and should be incorporated into the interview question list to some degree.[19]

Encourage existing employees to refer qualified candidates. Employee referral programs can be effective in sourcing candidates who align with your organization's culture and values. Consider offering incentives to employees who refer successful hires.

Retention Strategies

Employee retention is even more vital to your success than recruitment as the knowledge of your organization, processes, provider and patients leaves with them. Additionally, according to an article from Oracle, the cost of replacing even one employee in healthcare can range from six to nine months of their salary (and even up to 200% of their total salary for a highly specialized employee or provider) due to the impact to patient volumes and overall team productivity.[20]

Compensation is a key component of an organization's retention strategy to ensure team members feel fairly compensated for their roles and efforts. For both retention and recruitment efforts to be successful, a strong compensation strategy is crucial.

To that end, healthcare leaders should ensure the following items are in place:

- Regular Analysis of Market Salary Data and Adjustment Process to maintain market competitiveness, especially for any hard-to-recruit or high-turnover positions
- Consistent Review and Clear Adjustment Process to Create and Maintain Pay Equity
- Clarity and Consistency between Performance Review Process and Correlation to any Corresponding Performance-Based Increases (if applicable for your organization)

Ultimately, most employees do not leave an organization because of money drivers (or at least that is not what starts their search). Rather, they often start looking because of dissatisfaction with things that impact the rest of their work environment, how they feel supported and alignment with the organization.

One of the most critical things you can do as a leader is to work to build a thriving culture where employees feel recognized and valued. I believe most people, regardless of generation, want to understand their role in the organization, where the organization is trying to go and how they contribute to that success.

Additionally, I have found after reviewing hundreds of employee engagement surveys that there are two key drivers as to whether individuals feel engaged in their organization: 1) They feel that others are held equally and fairly accountable and 2) They have input and influence into how they perform their roles.

Exhibit 3.2 Five Elements That Drive Engagement[21]

Meaningful work	Hands-on management	Positive work environment	Growth opportunity	Trust in leadership
Autonomy	Clear, transparent goals	Flexible work environment	Training and support on the job	Mission and purpose
Select to fit	Coaching	Humanistic workplace	Facilitated talent mobility	Continuous investment in people
Small, empowered teams	Invest in management development	Culture of recognition	Self-directed, dynamic learning	Transparency and honesty
Time for slack	Modern performance management	Inclusive, diverse work environment	High-impact learning culture	Inspiration
A focus on simplicity				

Graphic: Deloitte University Press I DUPress.com

Engagement Strategies

Creating a culture of accountability, clear expectations and collaboration are essential to building a team that works together and partners with you as a leader to identify needed changes and drive improved results for your patients and your organization. Here are some components to consider that can help your organization achieve this environment and increase employee engagement and retention.

Emphasize an environment of open communication and constructive feedback. Regularly engage with your team through one-on-one meetings, providing constructive feedback and addressing any concerns. Encourage and act upon their input and ideas, demonstrating a genuine commitment to improving the workplace. One of the best ways to do this can be a simple brainstorming exercise.

Prioritize the ongoing professional growth of your team, and empower them through education. Provide access to training and continuous learning opportunities that expand their skills and knowledge. According to Adam Lewis, CEO and founder of Apploi, this can even extend to young job seekers looking for opportunities in healthcare, especially those interested in learning and advancing while doing entry-level roles such as nursing assistants.[22] This investment in staff development not only enhances their capabilities but also signals the organization's commitment to their career progression.

There is a difference between losing a strong employee and losing one that is not contributing to the future growth of your organization. One of the quickest ways to have your high-performers leave is to see you tolerate one that is either under-performing from a productivity perspective or exhibiting negative behaviors that go against your culture or core expectations. Subsequently, it is critical to directly address under-performers. To increase your odds of having an engaged team and minimal turnover, you need to have clear expectations for the organization as well as individual roles so team members and your leaders know what success looks like. Then you must have a consistent performance management system in place to help your leaders monitor and address under-performers.

Outline transparent career advancement paths within your organization. Develop progression plans that detail the steps needed for professional growth, supplemented by mentorship and coaching opportunities.

Work-life balance can more accurately be described as work-life integration, which begins with acknowledging the critical importance of both the professional and personal lives of every team member. According to the Tallahassee Memorial Healthcare group, an unbalanced work-life mix creates stress and can lead to emotional exhaustion or burnout.[23] Leading and encouraging conversations that allow employees, leaders and providers to share what is most important to them in and out of the office can go a long way towards establishing trust and a partnership of how to build roles and strategies that support both as much as possible. This may include options like flexible scheduling and remote work options when possible or working on processes to ensure more predictable workdays so team members can make their outside commitments more often. Additionally, implementing programs that support the mental and physical health of your team, such as wellness initiatives and stress management resources, including employee assistance programs (EAPs), can help your team feel supported and cared for as a whole person and not merely their core job function.

Create structures to regularly obtain insight from your team. Regularly conduct employee and provider engagement surveys to understand the team's morale and engagement levels. Additionally, incorporate exit interviews into your offboarding processes to gain insights into why employees leave. Use these insights to identify and address areas needing improvement, particularly in terms of workplace culture and leadership practices, and identify any underlying issues causing turnover.

Recognize and reward top-performing employees to foster a culture of excellence.[24] Implement a structured recognition program that acknowledges outstanding achievements. Rewards can include monetary bonuses, additional paid time off, or opportunities for career advancement.

Chapter 3: Staffing and Operations

Diversity within the healthcare workforce is essential for providing culturally competent care and driving innovation. Leaders should actively promote diversity in recruitment efforts and create an inclusive environment where individuals from diverse backgrounds feel valued and supported so they remain and grow in the organization. We'll dive more into this in the upcoming section on DEI.

Engage your healthcare organization with the local community to build a sense of purpose and pride among employees. Participation in community service initiatives and partnerships with local organizations can enhance your organization's reputation and foster a sense of belonging among staff.

And remember that succession planning is crucial for ensuring continuity in leadership roles. Leaders should develop a robust succession planning strategy through efforts such as mentoring, leadership training and offering stretch assignments. Such efforts can include taking on a project or serving as a committee lead. For key leadership roles, pursuing external training or executive coaching can be extremely beneficial in supporting these individuals for the next level of growth in the organization.

Remember that retention efforts are even more important than recruitment efforts. Ensure you are expending as much effort supporting, training and developing your current leaders, team members and providers so they are aligned with your vision and partnering with you to achieve results. Ideally, recruitment then becomes more of an expansion tool than the primary focus we are having to spend most of our time on.

3.5 Strategic Outsourcing and Automation in Healthcare

Outsourcing certain functions and embracing automation can enhance efficiency, reduce costs and maintain or even improve the quality of patient care. According to a recent MGMA Stat Poll, more than 20% of medical groups say they will outsource or automate their revenue cycle in 2024.[25] Leaders should carefully assess which functions can be outsourced without compromising quality or patient care.

Exhibit 3.3 RCM Outsourcing and Automation

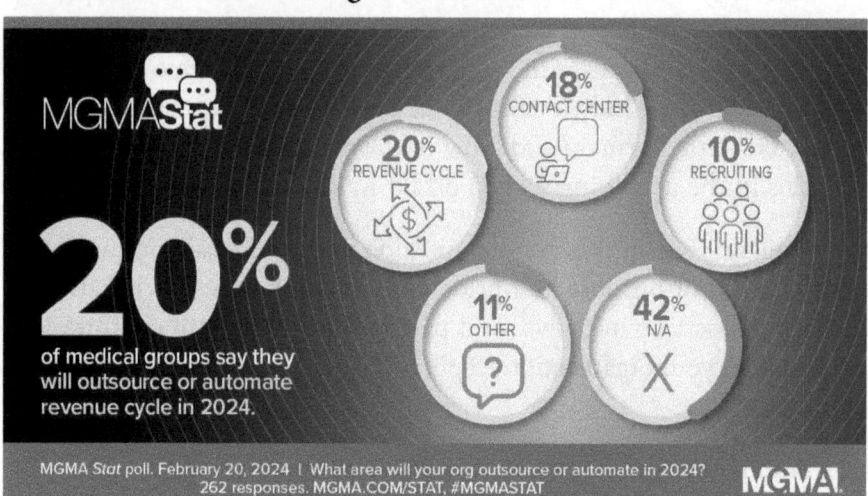

MGMAStat

20% of medical groups say they will outsource or automate revenue cycle in 2024.

- 20% REVENUE CYCLE
- 18% CONTACT CENTER
- 10% RECRUITING
- 11% OTHER
- 42% N/A

MGMA *Stat* poll. February 20, 2024 | What area will your org outsource or automate in 2024? 262 responses. MGMA.COM/STAT, #MGMASTAT

Evaluation of Areas for Outsourcing and/or Automation

A first step when considering outsourcing is to identify which non-core functions can be outsourced without compromising the integrity of patient care. This is where some of the process improvement tools such as process mapping and time observation/analysis can be helpful to define bottlenecks, resource needs and where outsourcing or automation best fit.

Vendor Vetting and SLAs: When considering an outsourcing partner, it is essential to vet them for compliance with healthcare regulations, data security measures and performance history. For each vendor and service being provided, it is important to establish service level agreements (SLAs) that define the expected service quality and reliability. An SLA might stipulate, for example, "Coding errors must not exceed x% of all coded transactions per month." It is also worth ensuring that outsourcing partners align with your organization's values and quality standards. Ideally, you are creating long-term relationships and many of these services will touch your customers directly so having alignment in key areas and approaches are crucial.

Quality and Impact Assessment: After implementation, it is essential to perform regular assessments to ensure outsourced functions meet quality standards and that the service is creating the desired impact from a process, financial and overall operational perspective.

Continuous Contract Review: Ongoing evaluation and renegotiation of outsourcing contracts can adapt to the changing needs of the healthcare organization. During these reviews, take the opportunity to alter and optimize key areas such as pricing, service and warranty components, feedback and training processes to ensure the services are supporting your evolving strategic goals.

Outsourcing Models

Outsourcing partnerships can range from fully outsourcing an entire functional area, such as your revenue cycle or scheduling services, or simply a portion of a process like prior authorizations. According to UK-based global outsourcing company BruntWork, healthcare process outsourcing focuses on optimizing essential but non-core tasks related to billing and coding, telemedicine, patient care and support services, and healthcare IT solutions.[26] It is very important to evaluate how the outsourced team members will interact both with your leadership team as well as your internal staff, providers and patients to ensure as seamless implementation and successful partnership as possible. Vertrical, a digital health technology firm, discusses the three main outsourcing models as they relate to healthcare:[27]

- **Offshore:** Offshore outsourcing involves sourcing talent outside the country, typically ones that are far across the globe. It can improve profit margins through reduced labor costs while widening an organization's talent pool. However, language barriers and conflicting work hours due to time zone differences can present major challenges. Plus, quality control can be difficult without ensuring the offshore team has sufficient standards and processes in place.
- **Nearshore:** Similar to the offshore model, nearshore outsourcing involves neighboring countries, often those within the same continent. Providing similar benefits to offshore outsourcing, the nearshore model makes quality control

much simpler thanks to closer proximity, as project managers and leaders have easier access to visit and communicate with their outsourcing partners. But because neighboring countries don't always speak the same language, many of the communication challenges from the offshore model are still present at slightly higher labor costs.
- **Onshore:** Simply put, onshore outsourcing is done locally within the same country. By eliminating most communication and logistical barriers, this model allows for much more fluid communication and quality control. Although this model effectively addresses the issues that the other models have, it is often the least cost effective. Oftentimes, it can be just as cost effective to hire in-house.

To determine the best outsourcing model for your healthcare organization, consider the pros and cons of each one as they relate to your organizational goals and values.

Automation

Automation in healthcare can lead to significant efficiency gains by streamlining repetitive tasks, enhancing accuracy and reducing labor costs. Leaders should identify processes that can benefit from automation. Consider implementing automation in areas like appointment scheduling, patient communication, prescription refills, and inventory management. It is worth noting that recent advances in AI have been penetrating the healthcare technology space at rapid rates and will continue to play an increasingly pivotal role in the industry, both in terms of outsourcing services and automating internal processes.

Here are a just few examples of how AI is being utilized in healthcare:

- **Diagnostic Imaging Analysis:** AI algorithms are being used to assist radiologists in analyzing diagnostic images such as X-rays, CT scans, and MRIs. These tools can identify abnormalities and help prioritize patient cases for review.
- **Virtual Health Assistants:** AI-powered virtual assistants and even some automated "bots" are being used to triage

patient inquiries, schedule appointments, and provide consistent follow-up care, automating the communication process and reducing the need for administrative staff. Fran Saperstein, CEO for Phoenix-based Center for Complex Neurology, says virtual assistants have become an important part of her organization: "It has been pretty amazing in changing the way that our practice runs."

- **Predictive Analytics for Patient Care:** Healthcare systems are utilizing AI for predictive analytics to identify patients at risk of chronic diseases or readmission. These solutions can analyze vast amounts of patient data to predict health outcomes and suggest preventive measures.
- **Natural Language Processing (NLP) in Documentation:** NLP technologies are being employed to automate the transcription of clinical documentation and patient interactions. The technologies convert doctors' spoken words into structured electronic health record (EHR) entries which can make quality outcome data needed for MIPS and other measures easier to collate, as well as improve the consistency of data for billing and operational analysis purposes.
- **Pharmacy Automation:** AI is transforming pharmacy operations with automated dispensing systems that manage medication inventories, track drug usage patterns, and reduce dispensing errors, streamlining the pharmaceutical supply chain.

While automation can enhance efficiency, leaders should ensure that there are mechanisms for human intervention when needed, particularly in clinical decision-making and patient interactions. This becomes even more important with the onset of AI technologies that, although come with tremendous potential, need customization and monitoring to ensure they are meeting the intended goals and adjusting for changes in your organization and the larger environment.

Data Security in Outsourcing and Automation: With the increasing reliance on technology, data security is a critical concern in healthcare. Leaders must ensure outsourcing partners adhere to strict data security protocols and comply with regulations such as the Health Insurance Portability and Accountability Act (HIPAA). Additionally, it is essential to ensure proper encryption, access controls, and regular security assessments are in place as part of the strategy to protect patient and other proprietary information.

Outsourcing and automation should be subject to ongoing evaluation to ensure that they align with the organization's goals and deliver the intended benefits. Leaders should regularly review the performance of outsourcing partners and the effectiveness of automated processes. Feedback from staff and patients can provide valuable insights into the impact of these strategies. Consider the following key factors for a successful change management in implementing outsourcing and automation.

- Involve team members in the identification of outsourcing or automation focus and selection of vendor or partner.
- Clearly communicate the changes to staff and provide the necessary training to ensure team members not only understand their role and how to use the system or partner with the outsourced team but also the intended goals and communication and feedback pathways of the technology or outsourced group.
- Consider phased implementation, when possible, to allow for adjustment and refinement. Implementation could be phased in by different work units or perhaps different processes or patient groups, depending on the risks and benefits of each option.
- Continuously assess the impact of outsourcing and automation on operations and patient care. Ensure metrics and KPIs are in place to monitor and analyze the impact of the outsourcing and automation initiative on the specific focus area or process and organizational performance (as a whole).
- Celebrate successes: As Medical Economics says, InHealth, a major provider of specialized diagnostic and health care solutions, was able to save 21,000 hours of work per year

using automation to assist with onboarding, billing and revenue cycle management.[28]

Incorporating these strategies requires more than just a transactional approach; rather, it can be a transformational shift in how healthcare leaders manage and operate their organizations. Ultimately, it's about building a culture that embraces innovation and change while ensuring that patient care remains at the core of all decisions.

3.6 Diversity, Equity and Inclusion in Healthcare Leadership

Diversity, equity, and inclusion (DEI) are fundamental principles that should be a cornerstone of healthcare leadership. As leaders, we should strive to create cultures that foster an inclusive healthcare environment, where we and our organizations can truly benefit from the range of experiences, backgrounds and perspectives of all members of all teams.

Importance of DEI in Healthcare

Diversity, equity and inclusion are integral to healthcare leadership for several reasons. Diverse healthcare teams can better understand and address the unique needs and preferences of a diverse patient population. This leads to better patient-centered care and improved health outcomes. Patients who see their identities and experiences reflected in their healthcare providers often feel more at ease and trusting in their plan of care once again contributing to improved health outcomes. According to the Harvard Medical School, healthcare inequity is a longstanding issue that medical providers may be able to help correct by recognizing those inequities and working to reduce disparities, to help improve the health of minority patients.[29]

Diverse teams bring varied perspectives and experiences, fostering creativity and innovation in healthcare solutions and practices. An inclusive work environment where all employees feel valued and heard leads to higher levels of employee engagement and job satisfaction. A commitment to DEI in healthcare leadership also builds trust within the community, especially among underserved populations, and can lead to increased healthcare access and utilization.

Strategies for Promoting DEI

With ongoing national debate about the merits of DEI practices in both education and business, healthcare leaders need to take proactive steps in ensuring the benefits and advantages of diversity efforts are realized and long-lasting. This begins by actively recruiting and hiring individuals from diverse backgrounds. Implement blind recruitment techniques to minimize bias during the selection process. As mentioned earlier in the section on recruitment, consistency throughout the hiring process is key to ensuring all candidates are considered for their unique skills and you are taking steps to build a diverse team.

Healthcare leaders should champion and model inclusive behaviors. Encourage open dialogue and ensure that diverse voices are heard at all levels of the organization. This includes a focus on training and education regarding diversity issues such as unconscious bias, cultural competency and inclusive leadership to staff at all levels.[30] Education is a critical component of building an inclusive culture. Healthcare organizations should also establish Employee Resource Groups (ERGs) that focus on different aspects of diversity such as race, gender, LGBTQ+ identities, age and disability. ERGs provide a platform for employees to connect and contribute to an inclusive workplace.

Collect and analyze demographic data on employees and patients to identify disparities and areas for improvement. Use this data to inform DEI initiatives and track progress. Finally, to promote equity in care, ensure equitable access to healthcare services regardless of patients' backgrounds or socioeconomic status. Putting in place both analytics that assess current disparities in health outcomes and actively pursuing initiatives that address them is very important for leaders to consider for ensuring they are providing culturally competent care.

Chapter 3: Staffing and Operations

Leadership's Role in DEI

As a healthcare leader, your role in promoting DEI is pivotal. According to Press Ganey, employees' intent to stay with a healthcare organization is increasingly associated with how they perceive the value their employer, manager and peers place on the presence and treatment of people from different backgrounds.[31] Here are a few actions you can take as well as encourage others across your team to continue to champion this important goal.

- Lead by example, hold yourself accountable for creating an inclusive culture, and champion diversity at all levels of your organization.
- Engage in ongoing self-awareness and education to better understand the challenges and experiences of individuals from diverse backgrounds.
- Encourage open and respectful dialogue about DEI topics within your leadership team and throughout the organization.
- Consider forming a DEI task force or committee to drive initiatives, set goals, and measure progress.
- Promote transparency in your efforts, communicating both successes and areas where improvement is needed.

3.7 Understanding Labor Law for Operational Leaders

Labor laws play a significant role in healthcare operations, affecting everything from employment contracts to workplace safety. Operational leaders must have a solid understanding of key labor laws to ensure compliance and mitigate legal risks.

Wage and Hour Laws

The most common labor laws that leaders need to understand are those addressing wage and hour regulations, specifically including both state and federal laws that focus on:

Minimum Wage: Understand the minimum wage laws in your jurisdiction and ensure that your organization complies with them. Keep in mind that some states have higher minimum wage rates than the federal standard.

Overtime Pay: The Fair Labor Standards Act (FLSA) requires employers to pay overtime to eligible employees who work more than 40 hours per week.[32] Understand the criteria for exempt and nonexempt employees, as well as the calculation of overtime pay. It is also important to understand the role of contract labor as it relates to staffing and the frequency of using contract employees for many roles in healthcare has increased due to shifts in the labor market and technology.

Family Medical Leave Act (FMLA): FMLA was implemented to provide security for employees who face serious health conditions or are required to take time away for care of dependent family members.[33] Healthcare leaders must navigate the complexities of FMLA with care and ensure they understand eligibility criteria, such as employees' tenure and hours worked. They should ensure clear communication about FMLA rights and responsibilities, maintain accurate records, and balance staffing needs while respecting employees' FMLA entitlements under the act.

Correctly overseeing FMLA can be complicated, especially in cases of intermittent FMLA, which is where documenting time away as well as the impact of the absence and whether it can be accommodated based on the job requirements is very important. Additionally, leaders must stay updated on any legal changes to the Act and integrate them into organizational policies, ensuring both compliance and support for their teams' work-life balance. It is important to engage your human resources partners when these complexities arise to ensure things are being handled appropriately.

For all of these regulations, it is very important to maintain accurate records of employees' work hours, wages, payroll information, absences and any FMLA-related activity. Compliance with record-keeping requirements is crucial to demonstrate adherence to wage and hour laws.

Anti-Discrimination Laws

Operational leaders must also be well-versed in federal anti-discrimination laws that protect employees from discriminatory practices based on factors such as:

Disability: The Americans with Disabilities Act (ADA) prohibits discrimination against individuals with disabilities.[34] Ensure that your organization provides reasonable accommodations to qualified employees with disabilities.

Age: The Age Discrimination in Employment Act (ADEA) protects employees aged 40 and older from age-based discrimination.[35] Operational leaders should take steps to identify and address age-related issues in the workplace. This information can often be collected through employee exit interviews and even during employee and provider engagement surveys.

Race and Color: Title VII of the Civil Rights Act prohibits discrimination based on race and color.[36] Ensure that your organization has policies and practices that promote diversity and prevent racial discrimination.

Gender and Sex: Title VII also prohibits discrimination based on gender and sex. This includes protections against sexual harassment. Implement clear policies and procedures for addressing and preventing harassment in the workplace.

Religion: Title VII also protects employees from discrimination based on their religious beliefs. Accommodate employees' religious practices and beliefs unless they pose an undue hardship on the organization.

Exhibit 3.4 Recent Title VII Changes

Recent changes in 2023 surrounding Title VII of the Civil Rights Act in 2023 have important implications for healthcare hiring and operational decisions.

There are several key aspects to consider, many of which will continue to evolve over the next year or beyond based on the ongoing discussions with the Supreme and Local Courts:

1. Broader Interpretation of 'Adverse Actions' in Employment: The Departement of Justice (DOJ) and the Equal Employment Opportunity Commission (EEOC) have urged the Supreme Court to adopt a broader interpretation of what constitutes 'adverse action' under Title VII. This could extend beyond traditional actions like hiring, firing, or promotion, potentially impacting a range of employment actions such as lateral transfers or shift changes.

2. Impact on Diversity, Equity, and Inclusion (DE&I) Programs: A broader interpretation of Title VII could significantly affect DE&I initiatives in healthcare organizations. This includes race-conscious corporate initiatives like mentoring, sponsorship, or training programs that might be restricted to certain racial groups, or policies that partially select interviewees based on a diverse candidate slate.

3. Legal Risks in Employment Decisions Based on Race: Following the Supreme Court's decisions, healthcare organizations should be cautious about considering race in employment decisions, as it could lead to legal risks and potential claims of discrimination. This includes being mindful of using race-based quotas or preferences in hiring and promotion, as well as setting demographic targets.

4. Aspirational Goals for Diversity vs. Quotas: While race-based quotas have been illegal, setting aspirational goals for improving diversity has been a common practice. However, the recent decisions might place these goals under greater legal scrutiny, particularly if they are quantitative in nature. Healthcare organizations need to carefully balance their diversity goals with compliance with Title VII to avoid practices that could be construed as granting race-based preferences.

For healthcare leaders, these developments underscore the need for a careful review of hiring and operational policies. It is essential to ensure that all practices align with the latest interpretations of Title VII, particularly regarding DE&I initiatives and ma king employment decisions that could be perceived as discriminatory.

Given the evolving legal landscape, staying informed and consulting with legal experts is crucial to navigating these changes effectively.

Chapter 3: Staffing and Operations

Occupational Safety and Health Act (OSHA)

Operational leaders have a responsibility to maintain safe working conditions in healthcare facilities. The Occupational Safety and Health Act (OSHA) established regulations and requirements related to workplace safety.[37]

Key considerations for leaders regarding this include:

- **Safety Protocols:** Develop and implement safety protocols to protect employees from hazards associated with healthcare work. This includes measures such as infection control, handling hazardous materials, and safe patient handling practices.
- **Training:** Provide employees with appropriate training on workplace safety, including the proper use of personal protective equipment (PPE) and emergency response procedures.
- **Record-Keeping:** Maintain records of workplace injuries and illnesses as required by OSHA regulations. Promptly report serious injuries to OSHA as mandated.
- **Inspections:** Prepare for and cooperate with OSHA inspections. Ensure that your healthcare facility is in compliance with OSHA standards to prevent citations and penalties.

Understanding labor laws and ensuring compliance is essential for operational leaders in healthcare. It not only mitigates legal risks but also contributes to a fair and safe work environment for all employees. Operational leaders should work closely with their HR departments and legal counsel to stay current with labor laws and regulations. Regular training for staff on labor law compliance is essential to prevent legal issues and protect employee rights.

3.8 Practice in Action

An outpatient cardiology practice desired to enhance efficiency and patient care in their procedure rooms. One of the key factors they found were that the room set-ups were inconsistent and staff were often spending excess time finding and retrieving necessary supplies for procedures. They decided to start with a Lean Six Sigma-inspired "5S" initiative to drive change, improving processes by optimizing clinical flow and reducing waste. These five steps, adopted from the world of manufacturing—sort, set in order, shine, standardize and sustain—describe the physical steps taken to reduce process variation and standardize outcomes.[38] During the event, the team took the following actions:

Sort: The practice assessed and decluttered procedure rooms, removing unnecessary equipment and supplies to create a more organized environment.[39]

Set in Order: The team organized the remaining items logically, ensuring easy access to essential tools and resources during procedures. They established consistent locations for the items (drawer vs. cabinet, etc.) and set quantities of the supplies to be stored in each location based on how often each supply was used during the time period they selected.[40]

Shine: A rigorous cleaning schedule was established to maintain a sterile and safe environment, reducing the risk of infections.

Standardize: Standard operating procedures (SOPs) were developed for patient preparation, equipment setup, and post-procedure cleaning, ensuring consistency and efficiency. They also implemented a card system to clearly alert staff when they needed to retrieve additional supplies for the procedure room because they were running low and place these in the supply storage rooms as well to trigger the need to order incremental supplies.

Sustain: A culture of continuous improvement was fostered, with regular audits, staff training and recognition for maintaining the optimized procedure rooms.

Through the effort, the practice was able to achieve:

- **Reduced Procedure Times:** Optimized rooms and streamlined processes led to shorter procedure durations, improving patient flow.
- **Enhanced Team Experience:** The efficient setup and standardized procedures contributed to a smoother flow for staff

and providers as they were able to more quickly have what they needed where and when they needed it throughout the cases.
- **Decreased Supply Costs:** By being able to quickly locate items, they decreased the frequency of ordering excess supplies that had contributed to not only clutter but unnecessary expenses.
- **Engaged Staff:** Employees were excited by the organized and more efficient spaces and grateful for the reduced frustration time and decreased walking time, resulting in improved morale.
- **Sustainable Culture:** A commitment to ongoing improvement ensured the longevity of the optimized procedure rooms.

3.9 Summary

Leadership in healthcare is not merely a role; it is a calling—a calling to inspire, innovate and elevate the quality of care for every patient and the well-being of every healthcare professional. We have addressed many of the critical facets of healthcare leadership that drive transformative change. Properly planned staffing and operations management is especially important in keeping the practice moving with efficient, engaged and technologically-savvy employees, as well as retaining compliance with key labor laws.

- Monitoring key financial and operational indicators provides healthcare leaders with the compass to navigate the complex healthcare landscape. These metrics illuminate the path toward financial sustainability and the delivery of exceptional care.
- Traditional staffing models may no longer reflect current healthcare workload. Adopting flexible, team-based approaches and better integrating technology will help balance the workload and prevent burnout and turnover.
- Recruiting and retaining top talent is fundamental. By recognizing and rewarding excellence, supporting professional

development, and fostering work-life balance, healthcare leaders can build teams that are resilient and driven.
- Outsourcing and automation can enhance efficiency and reduce costs. But that technology should always serve the ultimate goal—providing the best possible patient care.
- The world of healthcare leadership is richer and more impactful when diversity, equity, and inclusion are embraced. Commitment to these principles makes for better leaders capable of delivering equitable care and driving innovation.
- Navigating the intricate landscape of labor laws is not just a legal obligation but also a moral one. By upholding fair and just practices, healthcare leaders can ensure that their organizations thrive as ethical beacons.

In the next chapter, we will examine current and emerging models for physician recruitment, remuneration and retention, including employed, independent and owner-operator physicians, as well as the opportunities created by remote work and telehealth medicine.

Notes

1. Amwins. https://www.amwins.com/resources-insights/article/the-importance-of-healthcare-staffing--ensuring-quality-care-and-mitigating-risks
2. IFEBP. https://blog.ifebp.org/benefits-percentage-of-payroll/
3. Academy to Innovate HR. https://www.aihr.com/blog/productivity-metrics/
4. Physicians Thrive. https://physiciansthrive.com/physician-compensation/wrvu-physician-compensation/
5. MGMA. https://www.mgma.com/datadive/practice-operations
6. CDC. https://www.cdc.gov/workplacehealthpromotion/initiatives/resource-center/case-studies/engaging-employees.html
7. DropStat. https://dropstat.com/blog/employee-scheduling/predictive-analytics-in-healthcare/
8. Marquee Staffing. https://www.marqueestaffing.com/2023/05/26/the-importance-of-adequate-staffing-in-healthcare/
9. AAMC. https://www.aamc.org/news/press-releases/aamc-report-reinforces-mounting-physician-shortage

Chapter 3: Staffing and Operations

10. MGMA. https://www.mgma.com/articles/staffing-to-demand-how-a-medical-group-illuminated-staffing-needs
11. ShiftMed. https://www.shiftmed.com/blog/the-role-of-ai-in-healthcare-staffing-enhancing-efficiency-and-accuracy/
12. Insight Software. https://insightsoftware.com/blog/25-best-healthcare-kpis-and-metric-examples/
13. AMA. https://www.ama-assn.org/system/files/steps-forward-private-practice-staffing-guide.pdf
14. American Nurse Journal. https://www.myamericannurse.com/patient-centered-staffing-as-the-path-forward/
15. Health Staff Group. https://healthstaffgroup.com/the-impact-of-telemedicine-on-staffing-needs-adapting-to-the-new-frontier-of-healthcare-delivery/
16. American Hospital Association. https://www.aha.org/workforce-strategies/recruitment-retention-strategies
17. KNB Communications. https://www.knbcomm.com/blog/10-tactics-to-build-a-strong-healthcare-brand
18. Kimedics. https://www.kimedics.com/blog/strategies-for-healthcare-talent-acquisition
19. Northeastern University. https://careers.northeastern.edu/article/interview-type-behavioral-and-situational/
20. Oracle. https://www.oracle.com/human-capital-management/cost-employee-turnover-healthcare/
21. Deloitte. https://www2.deloitte.com/content/dam/insights/us/articles/employee-engagement-strategies
22. Forbes. https://www.forbes.com/sites/forbesbusinesscouncil/2021/09/08/four-ways-to-increase-hiring-opportunities-and-retention-in-the-healthcare-industry/?sh=1dab6c13f07d
23. Tallahassee Memorial Healthcare. https://www.tmh.org/healthy-living/blogs/healthy-living/colleague-stories-finding-work-life-balance-in-healthcare
24. Nectar HR. https://nectarhr.com/blog/healthcare-employee-recognition-programs
25. MGMA. https://www.mgma.com/mgma-stat/revenue-recruiting-and-patients-3-key-areas-of-outsourcing-automation
26. BruntWork. https://www.bruntwork.co/healthcare-outsourcing-trends-and-practices/
27. Vertrical. https://vertrical.com/en-US/blog/whats-the-best-outsourcing-model-for-healthcare-technologies
28. MGMA. https://www.mgma.com/mgma-stats/outsourcing-automation-may-provide-help-to-short-staffed-practices
29. HHS. https://www.hhs.gov/hipaa/index.html

30. Medical Economics. https://www.medicaleconomics.com/view/how-ai-powered-automation-supports-health-care-workers-and-improves-patient-care
31. Harvard Medical School. https://corporatelearning.hms.harvard.edu/blog/why-health-care-companies-should-walk-walk-when-comes-dei
32. American Hospital Association. https://www.aha.org/workforce-strategies/diversity-equity-inclusion
33. Press Ganey. https://info.pressganey.com/press-ganey-blog-healthcare-experience-insights/why-healthcare-diversity-and-equity-are-central-to-employee-retention
34. DOL. https://www.dol.gov/general/topic/workhours/overtime
35. DOL. https://www.dol.gov/agencies/whd/fmla
36. ADA. https://www.ada.gov/
37. DOL. https://www.dol.gov/general/topic/discrimination/agedisc
38. Federal Trade Commission. https://www.ftc.gov/policy-notices/no-fear-act/protections-against-discrimination
39. OSHA. https://www.osha.gov/laws-regs/oshact/completeoshact
40. MGMA. https://www.mgma.com/articles/5s-your-practice-for-optimal-success

Chapter 4

Current and Emerging Physicians Models

By: Jessica Minesinger,
CMOM, CMPE, FACMPE

4.1 Introduction

There is an expression that goes, "If you've seen one, then you've seen them all." This applies to some things in life, but not physician compensation models and employment structures. At an MGMA Annual Meeting, a speaker once said, "If you've seen one Physician Employment Agreement Compensation Plan… you've seen one Physician Employment Agreement and Compensation Plan." Engaging and retaining physicians is a critical aspect of healthcare management, and various employment models have emerged to address the unique needs and preferences of different types of physicians at different stages of their lives and careers.

This chapter provides an overview of current and emerging models for engaging physicians, focusing on the employed physician, independent physician, owner-operator physician, Independent Practice Associations (IPAs) and other emerging models, including remote work and telehealth.

4.2 Challenges of Physician Engagement and Retention

The U.S. is experiencing a shortage of physicians across most specialties. The demand for healthcare services continues to rise, driven by factors such as an aging and growing population, advances in AI and technology, and increased access to healthcare due to a labor shortage and state and national policy changes. Physician shortages exacerbate both the retention challenge and burnout as organizations struggle to maintain adequate staffing levels. Given these challenges, flexibility and agility in navigating physician employment models are crucial for recruiting, retaining, and engaging physicians.

According to an April 4, 2023, MGMA Stat Poll, among practice leaders who did not add new part-time or flexible-schedule physician roles, the prospect of hiring for nontraditional roles in the future depended largely on:[1]

- Whether looming retirements come from hard-to-recruit specialties
- Physical space limitations within existing facilities
- Being able to do part-time in the given specialty and take equal call
- The economic costs of onboarding and credentialing versus the lower revenue creation of part-time physicians
- Determining whether staffing models could be adjusted to add more clinical support staff for existing physicians, including part-time and flexible-schedule physician assistant (PA) and nurse practitioner (NP) positions.

In a 2023 MGMA webinar, "Thinking Outside the Box: Creative Physician Recruiting for Hard-to-Fill Positions," Tara Osseck, MHA, and Neil Waters, both regional vice presidents of recruiting at Jackson Physician Search, detailed the new approaches that help secure the right candidates amid growing competition for a shrinking supply of physicians.[2]

They note that about two in five physicians will reach retirement age in the next 10 years, but that residency slots are mostly stagnant despite increasing medical school enrollments. Finding the right solutions to new physician recruitment should consider the costs of losing a key physician without a replacement lined up.

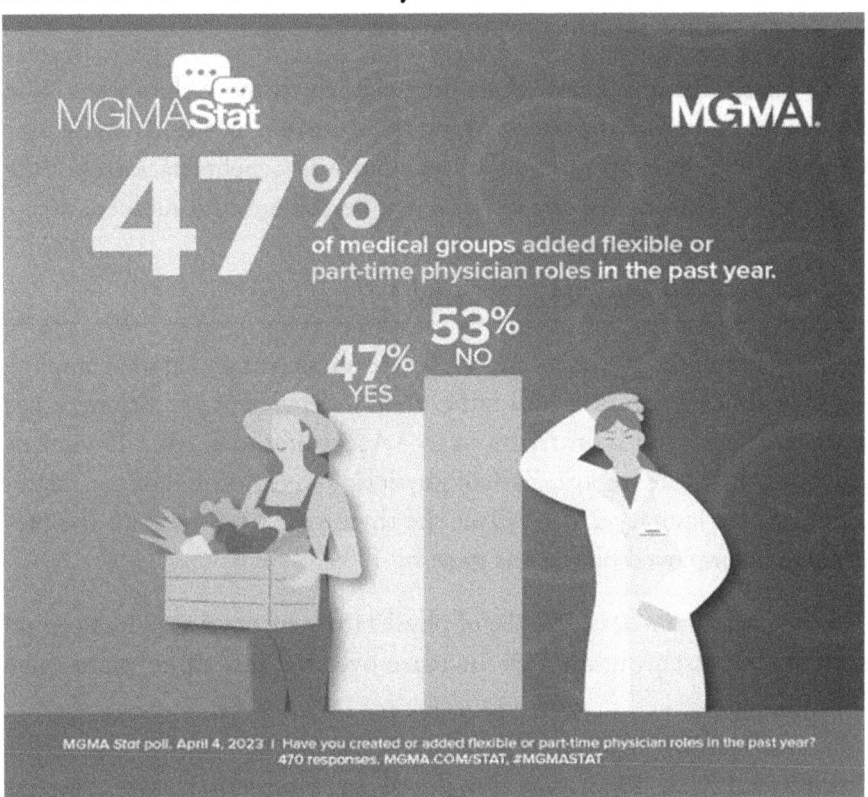

Chapter 4: Current and Emerging Physicians Models

Exhibit 4.1 Flexible/Part-Time Physician Roles Added

MGMAStat — MGMA

47% of medical groups added flexible or part-time physician roles in the past year.

47% YES 53% NO

MGMA Stat poll, April 4, 2023. | Have you created or added flexible or part-time physician roles in the past year? 470 responses. MGMA.COM/STAT, #MGMASTAT

"The estimated lost revenue for a noninvasive cardiologist opening that sits vacant for six months is about $1.15 million," Osseck said. "A gastroenterology vacancy sitting open for the same amount of time is about $1.4 million. ... An ophthalmology vacancy is the equivalent of $1.6 million in lost revenue."

When it comes time to fill a vacancy, Osseck noted that the industry average across all specialties is around the six-month mark, but that in the most competitive specialties or most-difficult-to-recruit regions, it might need an additional six months to fill a physician vacancy.

Beyond the lost revenue of physician vacancies, there are other major implications such as: lost market share, the effect of burnout on other physicians and providers trying to make up for the vacancy, and added

77

costs from using a locum tenens provider, Osseck added, while the search for a permanent replacement is underway.

"Physicians now know their financial worth more than ever...and they're deciding for themselves how their current positions stack up," Osseck noted, by examining offers for improved benefits packages or the promise of a better work-life balance in a flexible scheduling scenario.

4.3 Employed Physician Model

The employed physician model, where physicians are salaried employees of healthcare organizations rather than independent practitioners, has increased significantly in recent years.[3] According to a 2022 Physicians Advocacy Institute Report, 74% of physicians were hospital or corporate-employed by January 2022.[4] Over the three-year study period, the percentage of employed physicians grew by 19%.

As of January 2022, 52.1% of physicians were employed by hospital systems, representing an 11% increase over the last three years since 2020.

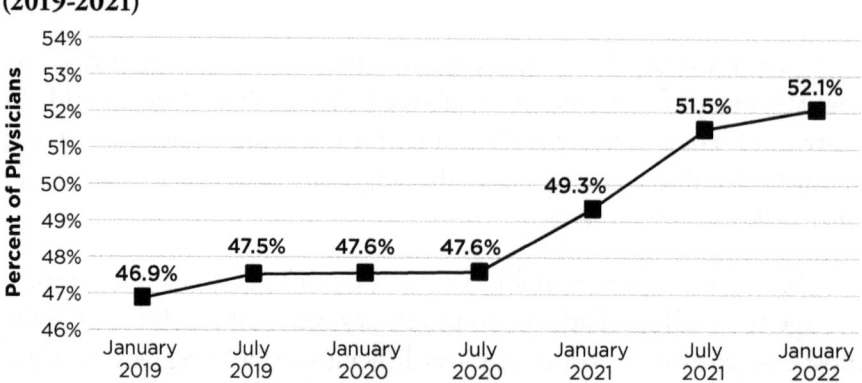

Exhibit 4.2 U.S. Physicians Employed by Hospitals/Health Systems (2019-2021)

Date	Percent of Physicians
January 2019	46.9%
July 2019	47.5%
January 2020	47.6%
July 2020	47.6%
January 2021	49.3%
July 2021	51.5%
January 2022	52.1%

The study found that 21.8% of physicians were employed by corporate entities other than hospital systems, representing an increase of 43% over the same three-year period.

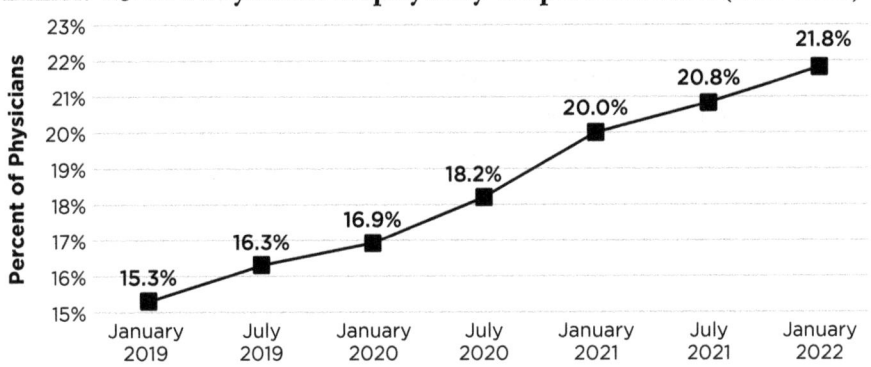

Chapter 4: Current and Emerging Physicians Models

Exhibit 4.3 U.S. Physicians Employed by Corporate Entities (2019-2021)

A line chart showing Percent of Physicians over time:
- January 2019: 15.3%
- July 2019: 16.3%
- January 2020: 16.9%
- July 2020: 18.2%
- January 2021: 20.0%
- July 2021: 20.8%
- January 2022: 21.8%

It's clear from the data that many independent physicians and physician groups were significantly impacted by COVID-19 and fled to the perceived financial safety of hospital systems and corporate entities. In fact, "nationwide growth in acquisitions of physician practices and employed physicians further accelerated in 2021 as the Pandemic continued."

As independent medical practices found they had lost leverage in negotiating reimbursement rates with insurers, many doctors went in-house at larger health systems, which could use their size to secure better deals.

The passing of the Affordable Care Act in 2010, along with federal rule-making efforts, rewarded bigness by tying reimbursement to certain health outcomes, like the portion of patients who must be readmitted. Getting bigger helped a hospital system diversify its patient population, the way an insurer does, so that certain groups of high-risk patients weren't financially ruinous. According to the *New York Times*, administrators have increasingly evaluated their medical staff according to similar metrics tied to patients' health and put a variety of incentives and mandates in place."[5]

The employed physician model comes with its own set of advantages and challenges. To effectively engage and retain employed physicians, healthcare practices must consider these factors:

Advantages

- **Stable and predictable income:** Employed physicians often receive consistent salaries and benefits, providing

financial stability compared to the variable income of private practice.
- **Reduced administrative burden and costs:** Healthcare organizations typically handle administrative tasks such as billing, coding and staffing, allowing physicians to focus more on patient care.
- **Access to resources:** Employed physicians often have access to more modern facilities, equipment, technology and support staff, which can enhance patient care.
- **Shared risk:** In some cases, the risk is shared between the physician and the organization, particularly in value-based care models, reducing financial pressures on individual physicians.
- **Career advancement:** Opportunities and protected time for career growth, such as leadership roles and involvement in research, may be more readily available within healthcare organizations.

Challenges

- **Loss of autonomy:** Employed physicians may have less autonomy in decision-making than independent practitioners. This is especially true as healthcare systems merge, which can frustrate some physicians.
- **Productivity pressure:** Healthcare organizations may have productivity expectations that pressure physicians to see a certain number of patients or generate revenue, which can lead to burnout.
- **Complex employment agreements:** Employment contracts can be complicated and may have non-compete clauses or restrictions limiting a physician's ability to practice elsewhere.
- **Integration challenges:** Integrating employed physicians into the culture and workflows of the organization can be challenging, especially if there is resistance from existing staff.

- **Financial uncertainty:** While employed physicians have a predictable salary, they may have less potential for high earnings compared to private practice, particularly if the organization's financial performance is poor.

In my experience working with both healthcare organizations and individual physicians, the vast majority of whom are operating or working within an employed physician setting, as organizations continue to see extraordinary growth, expansion, and mergers, making their workplaces feel personal and intimate is becoming increasingly difficult. By their nature, institutions are impersonal, and it can be increasingly difficult to make people feel a part of the system where they are empowered and have ownership. Physicians want to provide excellent patient care, make a positive difference in the world, and feel their input and contributions are valued and seen by their employers.

4.4 Engaging and Retaining Employed Physicians

Engaging and retaining employed physicians can be incredibly challenging in these larger, more consolidated systems. As Sachin H. Jain, MD, writes in a 2023 Forbes article:

"Much has been made about the problem of burnout. Recent findings published in Mayo Clinic Proceedings show that 63% of physicians are experiencing burnout. Just 30% say they're happy with their work-life balance. These numbers, of course, aren't entirely surprising. Highly educated, rigorously trained men and women who sought joy and career fulfillment through interactions with patients increasingly find themselves working for ever-larger, bureaucratic organizations where they spend hours each day updating electronic health records—the modern-day equivalent of 'paperwork.'"[6]

Healthcare professionals are prepared for hard work, Jain notes, but it is the nature of that work, and how they are treated by healthcare organizations, that feeds into burnout. Physicians and other healthcare workers say that their invisibility and lack of agency within an organization are critical issues, and that they often feel that their needs are being ignored.

Communication is Key

Engagement with physicians, then, becomes an issue of clear and consistent communication. Do not assume "no news is good news" if you're not hearing from your physicians. It's more important than ever to check in routinely. Communicate effectively, frequently, transparently and authentically. Physicians have identified two-way communication as one of their top priorities and expectations from healthcare leaders.

Effective communication is essential for understanding the concerns and needs of physicians. Healthcare organizations can employ strategies to facilitate open and productive communication, including:

- **Regular Feedback Sessions:** Implement regular sessions to gather input from physicians about their work experiences and challenges. This can help identify early signs of burnout and areas for improvement.
- **Physician Liaison Programs:** Establish liaison programs to bridge healthcare leadership and physicians. These liaisons can address concerns, relay information and build relationships.
- **Fostering Psychological Safety:** This is a crucial concept in high-performing teams that emphasizes creating an environment where team members feel safe, respected and comfortable sharing their thoughts, ideas, concerns and feedback without fear of negative consequences.

Strategies for Physician Engagement, Retention and Wellness

Developing strategies to engage providers may feel daunting and overwhelming. It's best to start with the basics. At the core, humans are motivated by or disengaged due to a hierarchy of needs. In *Managing with the Brain in Mind*, Dr. David Rock of the NeuroLeadership Institute writes, "One critical thread of research on the social brain starts with the "threat and reward" response, a neurological mechanism that governs a great deal of human behavior." [7] Neuroscientist Evian Gordon refers to this as the "minimize danger, maximize reward" response; he calls it "the fundamental organizing principle of the brain."

Chapter 4: Current and Emerging Physicians Models

Exhibit 4.4 Workplace Psychology

Although a job is often regarded as a purely economic transaction, in which people exchange their labor for financial compensation, **the brain experiences the workplace first and foremost as a social system**.

People who **feel fear, distrust, or unrecognized at work, limit their commitment and engagement**.

Healthcare Leaders who harness this dynamic can more effectively engage their Physicians best talents, support care giving teams, and create an environment that fosters productive change.

Promoting physician engagement, retention and wellness takes an intentional approach that is flexible, updated routinely and addresses the unique needs of each physician generation. To be truly successful, it must be an organizational priority and designed with physician input and buy-in. A more proactive strategy of recruitment and engagement can help better retain and reduce turnover in organizations that employ physicians.

This starts with more competitive and transparent compensation. Offering competitive salaries and benefits is essential to attract and retain talented physicians. As discussed in the previous chapter, promoting work-life balance through reasonable work hours, on-call schedules, and time-off policies can also help prevent burnout. Maintaining open and transparent communication with physicians is also important, addressing their concerns and involving them in decision-making when appropriate. Make it a practice to schedule routine check-ins with physicians consistently.

Other important initiatives include providing opportunities for continuing education, leadership development and career advancement. Continuing development can keep physicians engaged. Fostering a positive and supportive organizational culture that values physicians' contributions, diversity, generational differences, gender differences and well-being, will also demonstrate a commitment to physician health. This can be demonstrated by emphasizing the importance of quality patient care and providing tools and resources to support physicians in delivering high-quality care.

Finally, consider allowing more flexibility in practice to accommodate physicians' individual needs and preferences. It may also be helpful to develop and implement meaningful wellness program options, in collaboration with physicians, that promote their physical and emotional well-being.

A longer-term consolidation of healthcare organizations has left many physicians feeling as though they are powerless in extensive bureaucratic systems. When physicians feel they have at least some autonomy, decision-making discretion, and the resources available to excel in their jobs, they tend to feel less micromanaged and more fulfilled.

In summary, the employed physician model has its advantages and challenges. Healthcare practices can effectively engage and retain employed physicians by addressing these factors and creating a supportive and inspiring work environment that meets the needs of the organization as well as the physician.

Ultimately, at the very cornerstone of patient healthcare are physicians. Organizations that nurture and cultivate cultures of respect and genuinely engage physicians see better patient outcomes along with increased revenue, and are recognized as high performers.

4.5 Independent Physicians

Independent physicians, often referred to as solo practitioners or private practice physicians, operate their medical practice independently without being employed by a larger healthcare organization or hospital. Independent Owner-Operator physicians are responsible for all aspects of their practice, including patient care, administrative tasks, purchasing of equipment and supplies, coding and billing, human resources, and office management. It is an entrepreneurial endeavor with similar rewards and risks to running a small business.

Many physicians I've worked with prioritize hiring physician partners for the practice as one of the most critical components to running a high-performing, successful private practice. In addition to being clinical partners, these physicians are also business partners. This arrangement goes beyond employer and employee to financial partnerships. With more freedom and autonomy comes increased responsibility and reliance on your partners from a leadership and economic perspective.

In 2022, Physician-owned practices reported higher productivity levels in collections, total encounters, and wRVUs compared to their hospital-owned counterparts for 2022, according to the 2023 MGMA Provider Compensation Data Report.[8]

According to the AMA Policy Research Perspective—"Recent Changes in Physician Practice Arrangements: Shifts Away From Private Practice and Towards Larger Practice Size Continue Through 2022"—it found that between 2012 and 2022 the share of physicians who work in private practices dropped 13 percentage points, from 60.1% to 46.7%.[9]

"Importantly, those percentages include physicians who have an ownership share in the practice, as well as those who are employed in the practice (typically younger physicians) or contract with the practice," says the report, written by Carol K. Kane, PhD, director of economic and health policy research at the AMA.

The analysis found that in 2022:

- 44% of physicians were owners
- 49.7% were employees
- 6.4% were independent contractors

"This is in great contrast to 2012, when 53.2% of physicians were owners and, even more so, to the early and mid-2000s, when around 61% of physicians were owners, and the early 1980s, when the ownership share was around 76%," says the AMA report.

"When you look at young physicians today and compare them with young physicians from just 10 years ago, you see a dramatic change in behavior," Kane said in an interview, noting that the number of physicians under 45 who were owners dropped more than 12 percentage points from 2012 to 2022, from 44.3% to 31.7%. Established physicians, meanwhile, were much less likely to embrace employment as they moved through their careers.

Physicians in private practice may enjoy more flexibility and have opportunities for deeper relationships with patients and their communities. There is data to support that, for some specialties, self-employed physicians earn more than employed physicians. However, COVID-19 had a significant impact on physician-owned practices. MGMA's David Gans examined that impact in the following data study, conducted in 2023:[10]

"Provider compensation in physician-owned medical groups was much more affected by the changes in patient access and demand than was the compensation of providers in hospital-/IDS-owned systems. This is due to physician-owned practices functioning as independent businesses—the compensation pool available for their physician owners is the net of total revenue minus expenses.

"The data illustrates how surgeons and medical subspecialists were especially impacted by shifts in patient demand and the closing of ambulatory surgery centers (ASCs) and hospital operating suites. During 2020, operating revenue in most physician-owned practices decreased from the previous year, which lowered residual profits available to pay physician owners. Meanwhile, their peers in hospital-/IDS-owned practices were subsidized from revenues received elsewhere in their systems, reflected in the consistency in income levels during the pandemic."

Exhibit 4.5 Trend in Median Total Compensation for Selected Specialties

	PHYSICIAN-OWNED PRACTICES			
	2019	2020	2021	2022
Cardiology: Noninvasive	$468,506	$465,793	$500.441	$558,497
Family medicine (without OB)	$275,724	$288,107	$301,718	$309,263
Orthopedic surgery (general)	$581,044	$487.419	$619,942	$555.428
Surgery (general)	$445,137	$410,161	$474,191	$474,698

HOSPITAL/IDS-OWNED PRACTICES*				
	2019	2020	2021	2022
Cardiology: Noninvasive	$534,127	$530,500	$545,827	$559,839
Family medicine (without OB)	$252,296	$258,750	$262.483	$275.446
Orthopedic surgery (general)	$649,981	$661,923	$675,000	$684,699
Surgery (general)	$438,832	$446,262	$450,717	$472,570

IDS = integrated delivery system Sources: *2020-2023 MGMA DataDive Provider Compensation* (based on 2019-2022 data)

Figures 1 and 2 display the percent change each year in compensation and wRVU production for these specialties. The graphs show the direct effect of changes in wRVUs on compensation for the doctors in physician-owned practices, while the decreases in wRVUs during 2019 had relatively little impact on the compensation for the doctors in hospital-/IDS-owned practices.

The graphs also demonstrate the substantial decrease in productivity from 2019 to 2020 across all specialties and owners with the increase that occurred the next year that continued from 2021 to 2022. They reveal the volatility that occurred in compensation and productivity during the pandemic, especially for the surgical specialties.

Orthopedic surgeons in physician-owned practice reported a 16.1% decrease in compensation and a 9.8% decrease in wRVUs between 2019 and 2020, only to see an increase of 27.2% and 27.0%, respectively, in 2020–2021 but with decreases the next year. General surgeons in physician-owned practices reported a 7.9% decrease in compensation and a 12.6% decrease in wRVUs in the first year of the pandemic, with substantial recovery in 2020–2021 and only minor increases in 2021–2022.

Exhibit 4.6 Annual Percentage Changes in Compensation

FIGURE 1. Percent change in compensation and wRVU production in physician-owned practices

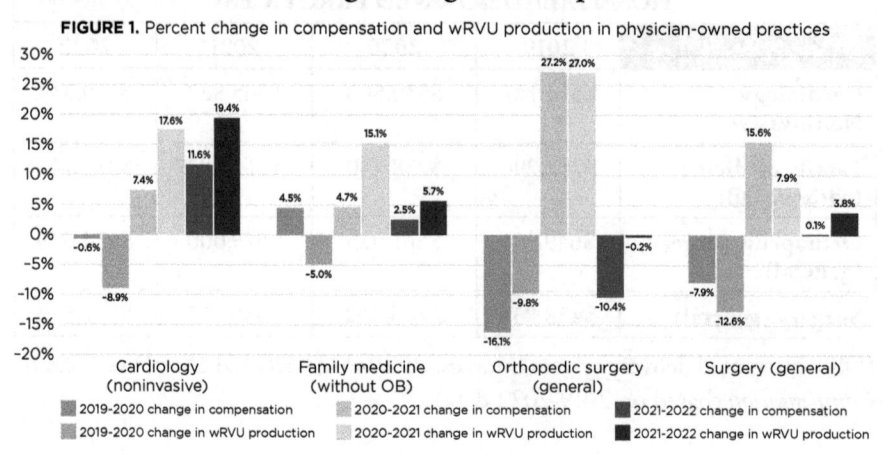

Specialty	2019-2020 change in compensation	2019-2020 change in wRVU production	2020-2021 change in compensation	2020-2021 change in wRVU production	2021-2022 change in compensation	2021-2022 change in wRVU production
Cardiology (noninvasive)	-0.6%	-8.9%	7.4%	17.6%	11.6%	19.4%
Family medicine (without OB)	4.5%	-5.0%	4.7%	15.1%	2.5%	5.7%
Orthopedic surgery (general)	-9.8%	-16.1%	27.2%	27.0%	-0.2%	-10.4%
Surgery (general)	-7.9%	-12.6%	15.6%	7.9%	0.1%	3.8%

FIGURE 2. Percent change in compensation and wRVU production in hospital-/IDS-owned practices

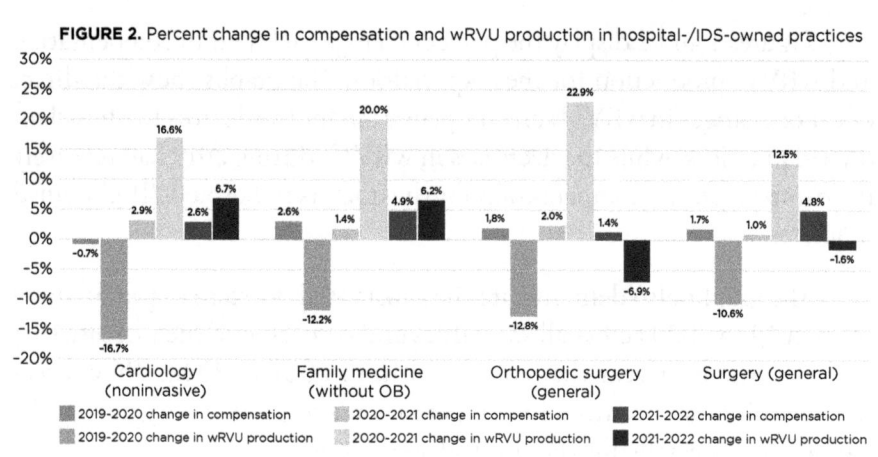

Specialty	2019-2020 change in compensation	2019-2020 change in wRVU production	2020-2021 change in compensation	2020-2021 change in wRVU production	2021-2022 change in compensation	2021-2022 change in wRVU production
Cardiology (noninvasive)	-0.7%	-16.7%	2.9%	16.6%	2.6%	6.7%
Family medicine (without OB)	2.6%	-12.2%	1.4%	20.0%	4.9%	6.2%
Orthopedic surgery (general)	1.8%	-12.8%	2.0%	22.9%	1.4%	-6.9%
Surgery (general)	1.7%	-10.6%	1.0%	12.5%	4.8%	-1.6%

The AMA study best sums it up regarding the "Pros and Cons" of Private Practice Ownership.[11]

- Empirical evidence suggests that physician-owned private practices deliver quality that is equal to, or better than, practices owned by systems.
- Leaders of high-performing physician-owned private practices are a distinct subset of physicians who place a high value on autonomy and independence in medical practice.

Chapter 4: Current and Emerging Physicians Models

- These physicians care deeply about their practices and the roles they play in their communities as healers and as small business owners.
- They tend toward feeling isolated, and many said they wished they had more contact with other like-minded physicians.
- Some physicians saw their only options as suffering under the administrative burdens and low payment rates or selling their practice to a larger entity with deeper financial reserves.
- Other physicians interviewed were driven to succeed. They were strategic in the way they managed change, adapting to value-based payment mechanisms, new technologies, and new practice models.
- Overall, the physicians we interviewed were highly professional and intrinsically committed to delivering high quality care.

They were also doggedly determined to succeed in private practice and very responsive to financial incentives and to peer comparison data when available.

4.6 Independent Practice Associations (IPAs)

Independent Practice Associations (IPAs) serve as intermediaries or networks that contract with both employed and independent healthcare practices, including physicians, to provide healthcare services to patients and financial and administrative incentives for physicians and practices. According to the American Academy of Family Physicians, IPAs offer many opportunities for innovation and can help to accelerate change in the way that healthcare is delivered.[12]

Pros of Independent Practice Associations:

- **Network Access:** IPAs provide a network of healthcare providers to patients, increasing physicians' access to patients to assist with sustaining and growing their practice.

- **Contract Negotiation:** IPAs often negotiate contracts with insurance companies and other commercial payers for their member practices. This can result in higher reimbursement rates and better terms.
- **Administrative Support:** IPAs may offer administrative support services, such as billing and coding assistance, which can help practices reduce administrative burdens, improve efficiency, and decrease time in accounts receivable.
- **Collaboration and Networking:** IPAs encourage networking and collaboration between member physicians, with the goal to promote best practices and improved patient care.
- **Collective Purchasing Power:** Negotiating collectively, IPAs benefit member practices in terms of cost savings and resources.

Cons of Independent Practice Associations:

- **Loss of Autonomy:** Participating in an IPA may require some practice standardization or adherence to specific guidelines, which could be considered limiting for some independent physicians.
- **Membership Fees:** IPAs often charge membership fees or a percentage of the reimbursement for their services, which can add to the operating costs of participating practices. The fees could be cost-prohibitive for smaller practices. Understanding the return on investment for each physician and practice is essential.
- **Limited Control:** While IPAs negotiate contracts, they may not always be able to secure the best terms, and member practices may have limited control over the negotiations.
- **Conflict of Interest:** Some IPAs may have a conflict of interest if tied financially to a specific hospital, network, or healthcare system. This could result in patient referral patterns or contract negotiations less beneficial to an individual physician or practice.
- **Regulatory Compliance:** IPAs must navigate complex healthcare regulations and may require substantial

administrative resources from participating practices to ensure compliance.
- **Changing Landscape:** The healthcare landscape is continually evolving, and changes in regulations, payer policies, or market dynamics can affect the viability of IPAs.

Professional associations, ACOs and IPAs can assist small and medium-sized physician-owned practices in contracting for network access that provides sustainable and competitive payment reimbursement. Physician practices also have access to industry advisors like attorneys, lenders, real estate experts and financial planners. The purchasing power of these groups can have a significant economic impact on purchasing big-ticket items like equipment, EHR systems and software, and other large asset purchases. These can be beneficial relationships if entered into with appropriate due diligence, including financial, legal, regulatory, market and demographic, and practice management considerations weighed carefully.

4.7 Emerging Models for Physicians

As further fallout of the COVID-19 pandemic, the opportunity for flexible physician work arrangements such as those offered by remote work models and through telehealth have given physicians additional flexibility—and may help incentivize others. Both models are significant changes from office-based traditional healthcare, but their benefits for both patients and practitioners has made them increasingly popular.

Remote Work Model

The remote work model for physicians encompasses patient consultations, diagnosis, treatment planning, prescribing and follow-up consultations from a location outside of a traditional medical office or hospital setting. Remote work can engage physicians and promote the retention of physicians who might otherwise retire or leave clinical work altogether. As evidenced by COVID-19, remote work models can be invaluable during public health emergencies, such as pandemics. Physicians can continue to provide care while reducing the risk of exposure to infectious diseases to their patients and themselves.

One of the primary benefits of remote work for physicians is work-life balance. Physicians can design their work schedules to align with personal and family needs, reducing stress and burnout, providing schedule flexibility, and increasing overall job satisfaction. Physicians who work remotely eliminate the need for daily commutes to a physical office or hospital, saving time and reducing stress.

Employers in remote work arrangements typically provide physicians with advanced telehealth technology and secure communication tools to ensure confidential, efficient remote care delivery. These tools facilitate effective patient interactions and accessibility to patient healthcare records. The remote work model can also significantly expand access to healthcare for patients, particularly those in rural or underserved areas.

Physicians providing remote work coverage who receive competitive compensation, including performance-based and quality-based incentives, stay engaged in remote practice long-term. Work arrangements may include administrative support for scheduling, billing and documentation, allowing physicians to focus their time on patient care rather than administrative tasks.

In an era of physician shortages that are projected to worsen and exacerbated by early physician retirements, an aging physician population, and record-high levels of burnout and turnover, the remote work model for physicians may prove to be a valuable tool to engage and retain physicians, while acknowledging and addressing the need for expanded, accessible healthcare services.

Telehealth Model

Telehealth allows physicians to consult with patients, diagnose conditions, prescribe medications and offer treatment plans without the need for in-person visits. According to Barak Richman, a Professor of Law and professor of business administration at Duke University's Fuqua School of Business, the lessons learned during COVID-19's experiments with telehealth suggest it is time to consider implementing those strategies on a permanent basis.[13]

"The 20th century model of healthcare delivery, in which patients get in-person care at designated brick-and-mortar facilities from licensed professionals, is reaching a turning point," he says. "Telemedicine, at-home care, and other delivery innovations—many of which achieved prominence when the pandemic struck—are offering new alternatives to hospitals, and data analytics are informing insurers how to better manage patients with chronic illness. Together, these innovations might forge a transformation away from a hospital-centric delivery system and towards an age of digital medicine."

Telehealth often provides physicians more control over their schedules and a better work-life balance. The flexibility of working from home, a telehealth center, a medical office or a combination of locations can be desirable for physicians seeking alternatives to traditional clinical and hospital settings. This increased patient reach can be engaging and fulfilling for physicians as they can serve more patients who might not otherwise have sought care due to proximity, affordability, or other barriers to providing healthcare services.

During the COVID-19 public health emergency, individuals with Medicare had broad access to telehealth services, including in their homes, without the geographic or location limits that usually apply as a result of waivers issued by the Secretary, facilitated by the Coronavirus Preparedness and Response Supplemental Appropriations Act, 2020, and the Coronavirus Aid, Relief, and Economic Security Act.[14] Telehealth includes services provided through telecommunications systems (for example, computers and phones) and allows healthcare providers to give care to patients remotely in place of an in-person office visit.

The Consolidated Appropriations Act, 2023, extended many telehealth flexibilities through December 31, 2024, such as:

1. People with Medicare can access telehealth services in any geographic area in the United States, rather than only those in rural areas.
2. People with Medicare can stay in their homes for telehealth visits that Medicare pays for rather than traveling to a healthcare facility.

3. Certain telehealth visits can be delivered audio-only (such as a telephone) if someone is unable to use both audio and video, such as a smartphone or computer.

Additionally, after December 31, 2024 when these flexibilities expire, some Accountable Care Organizations (ACOs) may offer telehealth services that allow primary care doctors to care for patients without an in-person visit, no matter where they live.[15]

Telehealth services are accessible, cost-effective, convenient and highly demanded. With new and expanded payment models, telehealth services can generate a consistent stream of patients and revenue for physicians and practices and, ultimately, be a flexible and viable financial option for healthcare organizations.

4.8 Practice in Action

Despite their best intentions, many hospitals have inadvertently found themselves with a mixture of employed and independent physicians, resulting in a complex management arrangement.[16] A Kentucky-based hospital had employed physicians, but was not a traditional group, given the following contradictory conditions:

- Primary care, specialist and hospital-based physicians under different tax identification numbers;
- Practices with dissimilar names and branding;
- On-site managers reporting to different hospital vice presidents;
- Billing done by hospital staff or by one of two separate physician billing departments on two different systems;
- Physicians on completely different compensation models and structures; and
- No group culture or feeling on the part of the physicians that they were a part of a larger unified physician organization.

A healthcare consultant was able to help create a separate entity for its employed physicians, as a subsidiary organization managed separately by a physician practice. Over a two-year period, new practices were added to the group, and existing practices transitioned into the new structure. A central billing office was established specifically for physician practice professional and technical services. An electronic medical record, integrated with the practice management system, has begun to be implemented in practices. Directors of primary care, specialty, and hospital-based practices were hired to oversee practice operations. The entity has its own Chief Administrative Officer, billing manager, credentialing coordinator and Director of Finance and Accounting. The practices have been branded similarly and are clearly identifiable as a part of the hospital's employed physician group. Physician compensation models have been implemented with similar values and structure.

Two years later, the hospital's employed physician group functions as a group, with better overall organization fueled by more accurate data and information, and a clear direction. The number of employed physicians at the hospital has also more than doubled, jumping from 27 employed physicians and a few advanced practitioners to a group of 64 employed physicians and 25 advanced practitioners. Medical coverage is provided in primary care, oncology, radiation oncology, general surgery, cardiac surgery, hospitalists, emergency medicine, urgent care, psychiatry and neonatology. The organization has also helped build the hospital's success by entering new markets with additional physician expertise.

4.9 Summary

These emerging employment models address various physician needs and preferences, such as work-life balance, financial incentives, reduced administrative burdens and opportunities for professional growth. Engaging physicians in these models often involves tailoring the work environment to accommodate individual career goals and lifestyle choices while providing the necessary support and resources to ensure quality patient care.

- A shortage of physicians across most specialties, plus an increase in demand for healthcare services driven by aging and a growing population, means it is more important than ever to focus on strategies to engage and retain physicians.
- The employed physician model has seen significant growth in recent years, providing more predictable income and

- reduced administrative burdens for doctors, but also less autonomy and more productivity pressure.
- Retaining employed physicians requires more involved and consistent communication, as well as a dedicated program of engagement and wellness efforts including flexibility and a supportive organizational culture.
- Independent physicians and physician-owned practices often report more productivity and revenue than employed physicians, and the high degree of autonomy and independence appeals to many.
- Independent Practice Associations can allow better network access, contract negotiation and administrative support, though there can be a loss of autonomy and control for individual physicians, as well as more challenging regulatory compliance.
- Telehealth work models allow physicians to practice medicine and provide consultative services while offering more flexibility, work-life balance and quality patient-centered care.

In the next chapter, we will look at strategies for physician workplace management, including physician retention and helping to prevent both physician burnout and turnover. These will also focus on measuring KPIs and improving communication to help promote better, longer-lasting working arrangements with physicians.

Notes

1. MGMA. MGMA Stat. https://www.mgma.com/mgma-stats/physician-shortages-forcing-medical-group-leaders-to-be-more-flexible-in-their-staffing-models
2. MGMA. https://preview.mgma.com/webinars/thinking-outside-the-box-creative-physician-recruiting-for-hard-to-fill-positions-on-demand
3. AHA. https://www.aha.org/system/files/media/file/2020/02/Market_Insights_MD_Ownership_Models.pdf
4. Physicians Advocacy Institute. https://www.physiciansadvocacyinstitute.org/Portals/0/assets/docs/PAI-Research/2022%20Avalere%20Employment%20Release%20-%20FINAL.pdf?ver=Cy6aAKaFlM56SND598Xlvw%3D%3D

5. New York Times. https://www.nytimes.com/2023/12/03/business/economy/doctors-pharmacists-labor-unions.html
6. Forbes. https://www.forbes.com/sites/sachinjain/2023/05/19/as-healthcare-organizations-get-bigger-healthcare-workers-feel-smaller/?sh=7d0f4ad06db2
7. Academia.Edu. https://www.academia.edu/13435526/Managing_with_the_Brain_in_Mind_by_David_Rock
8. MGMA. https://www.mgma.com/data-report-provider-comp-2023
9. AMA. https://www.ama-assn.org/system/files/2022-prp-practice-arrangement.pdf
10. MGMA. https://www.mgma.com/articles/data-mine-potholes-on-the-road-to-recovery
11. AMA. https://www.ama-assn.org/system/files/mathematica-ama-white-paper.pdf
12. American Association of Family Physicians. https://www.aafp.org/about/policies/all/independent-physician-associations.html
13. Politico. https://www.politico.com/news/magazine/2023/01/19/hospitals-competition-antitrust-00078393
14. US Congress. https://www.congress.gov/bill/116th-congress/house-bill/6074
15. CMS. https://www.cms.gov/newsroom/fact-sheets/cms-waivers-flexibilities-and-transition-forward-covid-19-public-health-emergency
16. HSG Advisors. https://hsgadvisors.com/case-studies/physician-employment-entity-infrastructure/

Chapter 5

Strategies for Physician Workplace Management

By: Jessica Minesinger,
CMOM, CMPE, FACMPE

5.1 Introduction

In the post-COVID era, healthcare is in the midst of significant transformation and one of the most pressing challenges it faces is the retention of physicians. The aging physician workforce, exacerbated by ongoing physician shortages, creates a complex landscape for healthcare leaders and organizations. Even younger physicians face tremendous pressures, which have led to an epidemic of burnout, depression and other mental health issues among the professionals patients turn to for their own medical issues. Others have decided to leave the healthcare industry entirely, seeking less stressful and more financially rewarding avenues.

In this chapter, we will examine some of the challenges related to physician retention, and take a closer look at the costs involved in coping with the disruptions of staff changes or prolonged shortages. By using appropriate KPIs and better addressing the reality of competitive physician compensation, organizations can work to help keep physicians better engaged, with a healthier work-life balance. They can also see the impact that four different generations of employees are having on the contemporary healthcare workplace.

5.2 Physician Retention Challenges and Impacts

Physician retention is a multifaceted challenge that healthcare leaders and organizations are grappling with.

Aging Physician Workforce

One of the most prominent issues in physician retention is the aging workforce. The baby boomer generation of physicians is approaching retirement age, and many are choosing to retire early, leading to a significant loss of experienced clinicians. As these physicians retire, healthcare organizations face replacing them with younger physicians with less experience, different priorities, and workplace expectations.

According to an August 2022 MGMA Stat Poll:[1]

- Before the pandemic and its myriad changes to healthcare, it was commonplace to see 6% to 7% of the physician workforce—approximately 50,000 doctors—change jobs or location.
- MGMA Stat polling from August 2022 finds that four in 10 medical practices (40%) had a physician resign or retire early due to burnout.

The data shows that aging physicians are most susceptible to early retirement. I've worked with physicians looking forward to retiring from their organizations only to turn to locum tenens work (temporary placeholder work). When I suggest that if they want to continue to work part-time, perhaps they want to talk with their current employers to see if it's an option, and more often or not, the thought hasn't occurred to them to ask, nor have their employers asked them. Recognizing the wealth of knowledge, experience and mentorship older physicians bring to healthcare organizations is essential.

Chapter 5: Strategies for Physician Workplace Management

In my experience, many physicians would stay longer if provided a flexible schedule, less administrative burden, mentorship opportunities, etc. Open communication is critical to determining what older physicians want and expect from their work-life balance. Retirement marks a significant life transition for most people, physicians included. Many are more comfortable with a partial retirement approach. They would be thrilled to work 2-3 days per week, run a clinic, mentor other physicians, serve on administrative and departmental committees, provide community education and outreach, etc. Outside-the-box thinking can go a long way to staving the mass exodus of physicians retiring; they bring tremendous value to our organizations that are worth saving.

An MGMA Business Solutions podcast with Tony Stajduhar, president of Jackson Physician Search, discussed the complex challenges of demographic shifts in the physician workforce.[2] Stajduhar said practice administrators need to start having open conversations with their physicians about their plans and why they want to retire. Understanding physicians better will help organizations better understand the options available to retain the doctors who might still want to deliver care part-time versus leaving the field.

"Let them know that you not only want to help the facility but that you also care about what they're looking for and what they need to make their lives better," Stajduhar said. "They're in a stage where life should be better and they should be able to transition and do what they want—they earned it."

Physician Shortages

The United States is experiencing a shortage of physicians across various specialties. The demand for healthcare services continues to rise, driven by factors such as an aging and growing population, advances in AI and technology, and increased access to healthcare due to a labor shortage and state and national policy changes. Physician shortages exacerbate the retention challenge and burnout as organizations struggle to maintain adequate staffing levels.

- Data from the Association of American Medical Colleges (AAMC) found that nearly half (46.7%) of practicing physicians were over 55 in 2021.[3]
- In other words, "more than 2 of every 5 active physicians will reach age 65 within the next 10 years."
- 40% of active physicians will reach 65 by 2031.
- The Association of American Medical Colleges (AAMC) projects a shortage of up to 124,000 physicians by 2034.[4]
- "If marginalized minority populations, people living in rural communities and people without insurance had the same health care use patterns as populations with fewer barriers to access, up to an additional 180,400 physicians would be needed."

And yet, given these challenges, a May 2023 MGMA Stat Poll found that only 15% of Medical Groups report having a formal program or strategy for physician retention.[5]

Exhibit 5.1 Formal Program Strategies in Medical Groups

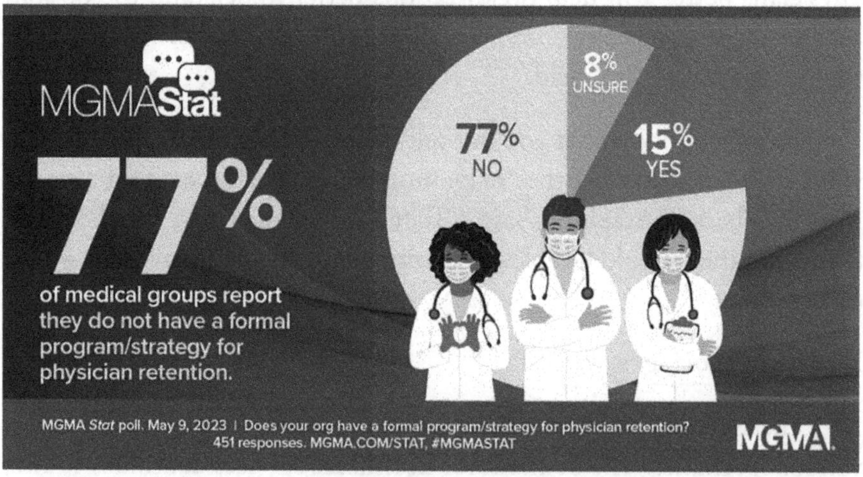

Additional market factors will likely exacerbate the physician shortage over the next 5-10 years. The tech world is increasingly appealing to healthcare workers who are burnt out and seeking flexibility in their careers. In a recent Healthcare Brew survey of 1,100 healthcare professionals, 70%

said they'd consider leaving the traditional medical field (i.e., hospitals, clinics, pharmacies) to work at a healthcare-centric tech company.[6]

The healthcare industry is already experiencing widespread staffing shortages. In 2022, 145,213 healthcare workers left the medical field, according to the latest data from healthcare analytics firm Definitive Healthcare.[7] Looking ahead, consulting firm Mercer projects that 510,000 healthcare positions may be unstaffed by 2026.[8]

Physician retention also directly impacts the quality and continuity of patient care. When patients can establish long-term relationships with their physicians, communication improves, physicians better understand individual patients' needs and quality and continuity of care improves. Physician turnover can interfere with these relationships, increasing the potential for errors impacting patient satisfaction and outcomes.

According to the American Medical Association, it has been shown in previous studies that less turnover and continuity of care between PCPs and their patients is associated with "better patient outcomes, including diagnostic accuracy, patient satisfaction, fewer emergency department visits, hospital readmissions, better care coordination, improved end-of-life care, reduced mortality and lower costs.[9]

Physician Burnout

According to the AMA, Physician burnout is a long-term stress reaction which can include the following:[10]

- Emotional exhaustion
- Depersonalization (i.e., lack of empathy/negative attitudes toward patients)
- Feelings of decreased personal achievement

Christine Sinsky, MD, AMA's vice president of professional satisfaction, shares, "While burnout manifests in individuals, it originates in systems. Burnout is not the result of a deficiency in resiliency among physicians, rather, it is due to the systems in which physicians work."

Furthermore, physician burnout is a major threat to healthcare quality, patient outcomes and the vitality of the medical workforce. More than half of US physicians report at least one symptom of burnout—nearly twice the rate of the general working population; many also experience depression, anxiety or suicidal ideation. Burnout is estimated to cost the healthcare system at least $4.6 billion annually, with the greatest burden attributable to turnover and work-hour reductions among primary care physicians.

Despite burnout's pervasive, wide-reaching negative impacts on our practices and organizations, a May 2021 MGMA Stat poll found that only 14% of healthcare leaders had a formal plan or strategy to reduce physician burnout.[11]

The Physicians Foundation's 2023 Survey of America's Current and Future Physicians finds that the state of physician well-being—for both current and future physicians—remains low.[12] For the third year in a row, approximately 6 out of 10 physicians often have feelings of burnout. Most physicians (78%) still agree that there is a stigma surrounding mental health care for physicians, while the proportion of physicians who report seeking medical attention for a mental health problem (19%) has remained stagnant since 2022.

Within the past year, nearly one-quarter (24%) of physicians know a colleague who has said they would not seek mental health support. Additionally, less than one-third of physicians (31%) agree that their workplace culture prioritizes physician well-being, declining from 36% a year ago. More than half of physicians (51%) know of a physician who has ever considered, attempted or died by suicide, remaining consistent since 2021. One-fifth (20%) know a colleague who has either considered, attempted or died by suicide specifically in just the past 12 months. Meanwhile, the portion of physicians who know the warning signs to look for in themselves or colleagues that may be suicidal (71%) decreased compared to 2022 (78%). Not only must we do better for today's physicians, but we must also help create a better reality for the physicians of tomorrow.

A significant challenge facing healthcare leaders is combating physician burnout and inspiring engagement and strong teams driven to provide the best patient care and outcomes. The positive news is that indications and data suggest that progress is being made.

Among the October 2023 poll respondents who indicated they had at least one physician leave due to burnout, more than half (55%) signaled that the organization has created or updated a strategy to confront clinician burnout in the past two years.[13] Those medical group leaders told MGMA that these efforts included:

- A shift to a four-day work week and the introduction of flexible work schedules
- Renewed surveys of clinicians to measure satisfaction, as well as the creation of physician wellness committees to plan and deploy burnout mitigation and prevention strategies
- Increased inclusion of physicians in wellness activities and resiliency counseling
- New emphasis on physician mentoring and coaching
- Offloading of administrative tasks to other team members, as well as improved training on enterprise EHR systems and implementation of enhanced tools to reduce technical burdens
- Use of hospitalist and part-time roles as a path to retirement for physicians who would otherwise leave

Still, not all respondents voiced optimism about ongoing efforts. In the case of geriatricians, one respondent told MGMA that the stagnation of Medicare payment rates is a unique driver of dissatisfaction and moral injury within the specialty. In other cases, the significant demands for patient care are difficult to balance with these efforts. Even as some organizations shift more of the workload to advanced practice providers (APPs), "there is no mechanism" available to properly combat burnout "with rising overhead and dropping reimbursement" adding pressure on physicians to work harder.

5.3 Physician Turnover Cost and Disruption

Implementing effective physician retention plans and strategies to reduce physician burnout is imperative to limit the financial impact and staff disruption attributable to turnover. The disruption is experienced by clinical and administrative teams who already may feel a lack of engagement and at risk of burnout.

Exhibit 5.2 Time Spent on Recruiting/Interviewing by Medical Group Leaders

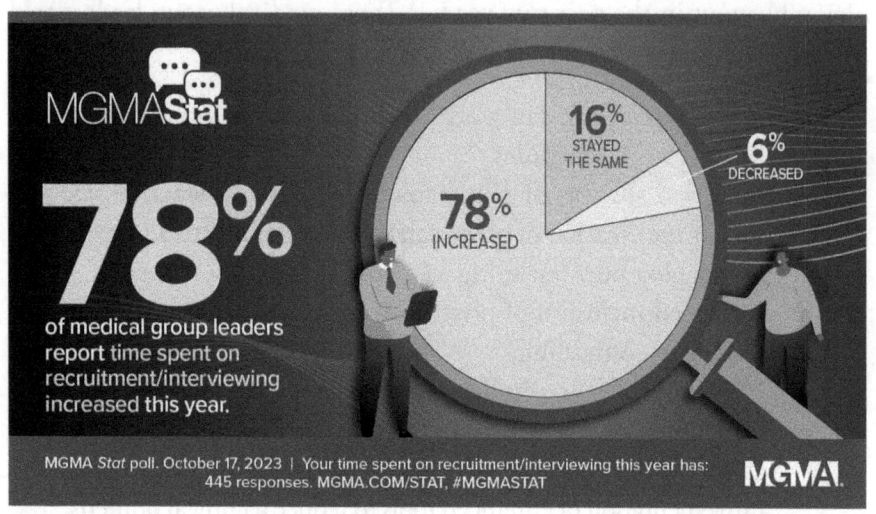

[MGMA Stat: 78% of medical group leaders report time spent on recruitment/interviewing increased this year. 78% Increased, 16% Stayed the Same, 6% Decreased. MGMA Stat poll, October 17, 2023 | Your time spent on recruitment/interviewing this year has: 445 responses. MGMA.COM/STAT, #MGMASTAT]

Physician recruitment represents a significant commitment of both time and money, with costs estimated at $250,000 per candidate, according to Jackson Physician Search.[14] Typical recruitment expenses include marketing and recruitment fees, candidate travel interview fees, sign-on bonuses, relocation allowances, tuition reimbursement, on-boarding, etc. The impacts of physician recruitment time are often costly and disruptive to organizations. The physician recruitment process is time-intensive, averaging 7.3 months to fill a family medicine position and 7.9 months for surgical subspecialties such as a cardiologist. These extended vacancies can result in substantial revenue losses, with medical groups potentially facing losses of $503,000 for family medicine positions and $1,607,000 for surgical specialists. The disruption to existing physicians in the wake of these vacancies further exacerbates burnout and turnover for the team.

It's no secret that having the right people—and enough of them—to operate a medical practice with optimized schedules is still the biggest roadblock to higher productivity, as noted in an April 2023 MGMA poll that ranked the issue of staffing firmly ahead of other challenges such as administrative burdens, patient scheduling and more.[15]

There's a common phrase that says, "activity begets activity." The same can be said for physician and staff turnover. The best-performing practices and organizations know this and prioritize investment in their teams, cultures and workplace environments, focusing on wellness, compensation transparency, engagement and retention.

5.4 KPIs: Measuring Retention, Burnout, and Turnover

Organizations must implement KPIs to measure retention rates, burnout levels and turnover rates to address physician retention effectively. Before developing a plan of action, measure where your practice is currently. The first step is to be honest with yourself and your team. Jack Welch once said, "Face reality as it is, not as it was or as you wish it to be." It may be conducting a SWOT Analysis (Strengths, Weaknesses, Opportunities, Threats), using Lean methodology to address challenges and benchmarking data to assess your unique strengths and weaknesses while developing comprehensive strategies to move your organization forward.

Measuring the state of the physician workforce and the effectiveness of physician retention strategies is crucial for healthcare organizations and policymakers to ensure adequate healthcare access and quality. Various metrics can provide valuable insights into these aspects:

- **Physician-to-Population Ratio:** This metric compares the number of practicing physicians to the population in a specific region or healthcare system. It helps gauge the overall availability of physicians and can highlight areas with shortages or surpluses.
- **Physician Vacancy Rate:** The percentage of open physician positions within a healthcare organization or region. High vacancy rates can indicate difficulties in recruiting and retaining physicians.

- **Physician Turnover Rate:** The rate at which physicians leave their current positions, expressed as a percentage. High turnover rates suggest retention challenges and can lead to disruptions in patient care.
- **Physician Satisfaction Surveys:** Surveys administered to physicians to assess their job satisfaction and overall work experience. Insights from these surveys can help identify areas for improvement in retention strategies.
- **Retention Rate & Length of Employment:** Average tenure of physicians within an organization or in a particular specialty. Longer tenures often indicate that current retention efforts are working.
- **Physician Productivity:** Metrics related to the volume and quality of healthcare services provided by physicians. High productivity may indicate effective retention, as satisfied physicians will likely be more productive.
- **Physician Burnout Rates:** Measures the prevalence of burnout symptoms among physicians. High burnout rates can lead to increased turnover, making it essential to address burnout as part of retention strategies.
- **Recruitment and Retention Costs:** The financial resources spent recruiting and retaining physicians. Monitoring these costs can help assess the efficiency of retention strategies.
- **Diversity and Inclusion Metrics:** Metrics related to physician workforce diversity. Measuring diversity can highlight areas for improvement in attracting and retaining underrepresented groups.
- **Patient Satisfaction and Outcomes:** Assessing patient satisfaction and healthcare outcomes associated with specific physician groups. High patient satisfaction and positive outcomes can indicate the effectiveness of the physician workforce.
- **Success of Mentorship and Development Programs:** Evaluating the impact of mentorship, career development, and continuing education programs on physician retention. Tracking the success of these initiatives can inform their refinement and expansion.

- **Exit Interviews and Feedback:** Gathering feedback from departing physicians through exit interviews. Insights from departing physicians can help identify systemic issues affecting retention.
- **Work-Life Balance Metrics:** Monitoring factors related to work-life balance, such as workload, on-call duties and schedule flexibility. Addressing work-life balance concerns can enhance retention.
- **Geographical Distribution Metrics:** Analyzing the distribution of physicians across different regions, specialties and healthcare settings. Identifying areas with shortages or surpluses can inform workforce planning.

By regularly assessing these metrics, healthcare organizations and policymakers can gain valuable insights into the state of the physician workforce and the effectiveness of their retention strategies, allowing them to make informed decisions to improve healthcare delivery and access.

Incorporating these crucial questions as KPIs for your practice or organization is an essential part of starting the process to address these challenges:

- **Physician Turnover Rate:** What is your Practice or Organization's current physician turnover rate?
- **Transition Planning:** Are physicians in your Practice or Organization preparing to depart or retire?
- **Retention & Burnout Plans:** Does your Practice or Organization have formal physician retention and burnout identification and well-being plans?
- **Plan Maintenance:** Are these plans routinely updated and adaptable?
- **Physician Engagement:** Are physicians involved in creating, administering, and updating these plans? Are they aware that the programs exist?

In his book *Think Again*, author and organizational psychologist Adam Grant writes, "If knowledge is power, knowing what we don't know is wisdom." [16] What you learn through searching for answers and asking questions will reveal the roadmap for your practice or organization to navigate and thrive in challenging and uncertain times.

5.5 Generational Differences in the Physician Workforce

Identifying and recognizing generational differences in the workplace—including values, motivators, communication and technology preferences, and work-life balance priorities—is essential to recruiting and retaining physicians. One size does not fit all, and navigating generational differences with openness and flexibility is crucial.

In her book, *Retiring the Generation Gap*, psychologist Jennifer Deal found in independent research that, "All generations have similar values; they just express them differently." [17] In other words, we might have unique ways of getting there, but we pretty much want the same things out of work.

There are four generations of physicians currently in the workforce, which include:

Baby Boomers (1946-1964): Baby Boomer physicians often value job stability and may be more resistant to technological changes. Healthcare organizations should recognize their contributions, communicate openly and proactively, and offer flexible work schedules and retirement transition programs to ensure a smooth transition.

Generation X (1965-1980): Gen X physicians are known for their adaptability and may appreciate leadership roles and work-life balance opportunities. Providing career development and flexibility can enhance their retention. They are known as the generation of "latch-key kids" who often had two working or single parents and grew up independent and self-sufficient.

Millennials (1981-1996): Millennials seek meaningful work and value work-life balance. Offering robust on-boarding, flexible and part-time schedules, telemedicine options, mentorship programs, and opportunities for community engagement can attract and retain millennial physicians. Communication, transparency and psychological safety are valued highly in a workplace environment. The latest generation to enter the workforce is:

Generation Z (1997-2012): The newest generation in the workforce, Gen Z, values innovation, AI and technology. This generation is described as resourceful and independent and highly values work-life balance. This generation can be skeptical of authority and often takes a "trust but verify" approach when presented with information.

Within the next few years, healthcare professionals will be expected to recruit, engage, retain and motivate four generations of physicians in the workforce. This indeed represents a challenge, but one that can be met with strategic plans, policies and procedures that are cognizant of and meet physicians where they are in various stages of their careers and lives.

And there are indications that healthcare organizations recognize the need and are moving towards flexibility. An April 2023 MGMA *Stat* Poll found that almost half (47%) of medical group leaders have added or created part-time or flexible-schedule physician roles in the past year, while 53% did not.[18] Medical group leaders responding to the poll told us some of the reasons for the updates to their hiring strategies:

- "Our older docs requested a more flexible part-time policy to help them keep working. Our old policy only allowed half- and three-quarter time."
- "To relieve some of the stress from an emergency call."
- "It provides the work-life balance that meets their needs or extends their retirement date further out."

So What Do Physicians Want? According to the Physician Burnout, Engagement, and Retention Survey conducted by Jackson Physician Search in partnership with MGMA in October of 2022, physicians seek the following:[19]

- 62% Two-way Communication with Management/Administration
- 57% Additional Compensation
- 47% Equity in Workload

- 45% Reduced Administrative Burden
- 35% Retention Programs

This is consistent with the feedback I hear from the physician clients I consult with. Open communication, clarity, and transparency regarding physician compensation are required to engender trust between physicians and administrators. Resist the urge to operate within an "us vs. them" mentality and focus on a "we" mentality that promotes solid, high-performing teams. When consulting with hospitals and practices, I recommend the following:

- Aim to create compensation plans that offer clarity and predictability.
- Physicians should clearly understand how their compensation is determined and the factors that influence it and have a sense of financial security.
- Avoid sudden changes or fluctuations in compensation whenever possible.
- Communication is vital to physician buy-in!

5.6 Physician Compensation

While it can be difficult to talk about compensation, it's important and necessary to physicians. We all want to understand how we are paid and to know that we are paid fairly. Physicians are no different. While many of us have business degrees and/or extensive experience in the healthcare business, most physicians do not. Physician compensation methodologies vary widely—compensation plans are often cumbersome and complex for administrators to administer, let alone explain. Meanwhile, provider compensation data—the predominant source for establishing physician compensation—is expensive, requires training to interpret effectively and is by no means easily accessible to physicians.

Physicians themselves are very much aware of wage and benefit discrepancies and have become much more active in seeking out better opportunities, especially since the COVID-19 pandemic. According to Physicians Thrive's 2024 compensation report, family medicine physicians earned an average of $255,000 in 2023, a 1.5% increase from the previous year.[20] Surgeons received a median pay of nearly $348,000 in 2023. Certain specialties also command top dollar, such as pediatric endocrinologists, who earned an average of $788,000 per year.

Equality in compensation is also a growing issue. According to the 2024 Medscape physician compensation report, despite an average 3% across-the-board growth in physician pay, male specialists earned an average of $435,000, compared to female specialists' $333,000 per year.[21] The organization's report also cited significant disparities in physician compensation between various racial and ethnic groups, with African-American doctors earning $37,000 less per year on average than white physicians.

Consider that 59% of medical practice leaders who reported better pay and benefits elsewhere were the top cause of staff turnover in 2021 in an MGMA Stat poll on February 1, 2022.[22]

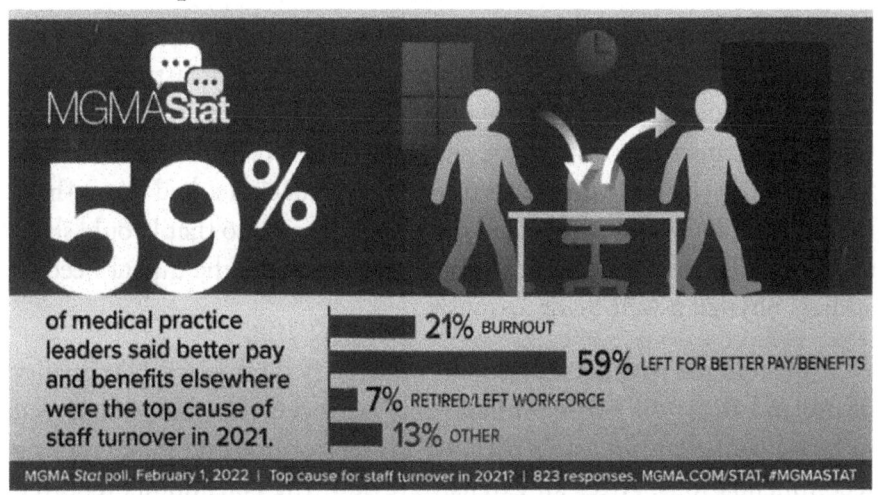

Exhibit 5.3 Top Causes of Staff Turnover in Medical Practices

MGMA Stat

59% of medical practice leaders said better pay and benefits elsewhere were the top cause of staff turnover in 2021.

- 21% BURNOUT
- 59% LEFT FOR BETTER PAY/BENEFITS
- 7% RETIRED/LEFT WORKFORCE
- 13% OTHER

MGMA Stat poll, February 1, 2022 | Top cause for staff turnover in 2021? | 823 responses. MGMA.COM/STAT, #MGMASTAT

Not talking with providers about their compensation and productivity along with not updating their compensation plans routinely to remain competitive can be costly for employers. So much of what happens is out of our control—this isn't one of them. Effective and routine compensation communication is a "best practice" that will pay off for your team and organization and is part of a thriving "we" culture. Exceptional leaders are eager to tackle problems, hear feedback and encourage those who dare to be honest and vulnerable.

5.7 Practice in Action

Addressing physician retention, turnover, and burnout proactively in your practice or organization is crucial to the success of your organization on many levels. I had just returned from presenting at the 2023 Association of Academic Surgeons (AAS) Fall Courses and the Association of Women Surgeons (AWS) Annual Meeting. I talked with physicians struggling to navigate their careers, compensation, patient care expectations, and work-life balance. These themes are familiar to me as a physician, practice consultant and independent MGMA Consultant. However, I am increasingly concerned about the depth to which the physicians I encounter are struggling and, to differing extents, suffering and considering leaving medicine early and altogether.

After a recent presentation, a hospital-based surgeon approached me to introduce herself. She shared that she was battling breast cancer. She told me unequivocally that her quality of life was better with breast cancer than before the diagnosis because she finally had a reasonable schedule at work and time for self-care. I was utterly taken aback. I asked her to share the circumstances at work that led her to feel this way so that I could share and hopefully inspire other healthcare leaders to take the urgent need to address physician well-being seriously.

She told me that her service was understaffed for years. Her quality of life and those on her team had been sacrificed. The hospital agreed to hire a consultant to assess the 10-FTE service line and make staffing recommendations. After an extensive review, the consultants reported that based on the volume, acuity of cases, panel size, trauma level designation, etc., the service should have 20 FTEs. The hospital unilaterally responded to the consultants' recommendations by hiring 4 FTEs, bringing the total to 14. To this physician, it felt like the consultant validated the team's concerns and made actionable recommendations; her employers acknowledged that their team was beyond over-extended "but didn't care enough to support the team to the extent that would fix the problem." She said the team's consensus was that they felt more hopeless and disrespected than ever. When diagnosed, she thought she finally had permission and the "justification" to scale back her hours and take time for treatment. I won't forget this story, nor the courage and vulnerability it took for her to share this with me. It fuels my mission as a healthcare leader to continue prioritizing and sharing the critical importance of physician retention, turnover, burnout, and well-being on our teams and the healthcare system.

5.8 Summary

Addressing physician retention, turnover and burnout is a complex but critical challenge for healthcare leaders. As the physician workforce and healthcare industry evolve, organizations must adapt by implementing effective retention strategies, measuring KPIs, understanding generational and gender differences, and fostering trust and open communication.

- An aging physician workforce is producing demographic shifts in healthcare management, coupled with ongoing physician shortages.
- Physician burnout is at record levels, as demands placed on a shrinking group of professionals cost the industry billions. Changes such as four-day work weeks, counseling, coaching and shared responsibility can help.
- The tremendous financial cost and systemic disruption of physician turnover suggests a more proactive strategy in retaining current professionals.
- KPIs can be critical in measuring the personal and financial issues related to physician retention, burnout and turnover. Metrics can help better engage physicians and create a better work-life balance.
- Four different generations are now at work in the American medical workforce, each with their own cultural needs, preferred communication style and working philosophy.

- Addressing accurate and competitive physician compensation can be the single most important factor in helping to keep doctors on the job, as long as possible.

By prioritizing physician engagement, well-being, communication and trust, healthcare leaders can successfully navigate these challenges and ensure the sustainability of quality patient care and the best possible outcomes.

In the next chapter, we will look at the various healthcare delivery and financial models which help to govern how a medical practice is paid for its services, and the revenue cycle management functions necessary to successfully process and close those claims.

Notes

1. MGMA Stat https://www.mgma.com/mgma-stats/burnout-driven-physician-resignations-and-early-retirements-rising-amid-staffing-challenges
2. MGMA. https://www.mgma.com/podcasts/business-solutions-how-to-prepare-for-the-wave-of-physician-retirements
3. AAMC. https://digirepo.nlm.nih.gov/master/borndig/9918417887306676/9918417887306676.pdf
4. AAMC. https://www.aamc.org/news/press-releases/aamc-report-reinforces-mounting-physician-shortage
5. MGMA. https://www.mgma.com/mgma-stat/finalizing-your-physician-retention-strategies-amid-worsening-shortages
6. Healthcare Brew. https://www.healthcare-brew.com/stories/c/state-of-the-healthcare-industry-hospitals
7. Definitive Healthcare. https://www.definitivehc.com/resources/research/healthcare-staffing-shortage
8. Mercer. https://www.mercer.com/content/dam/mercer/assets/content-images/north-america/united-states/us-healthcare-news/us-2021-healthcare-labor-market-whitepaper.pdf
9. AMA https://www.ama-assn.org/practice-management/physician-health/nearly-1-billion-excess-patient-costs-tied-physician-turnover
10. JAMA. https://jamanetwork.com/journals/jama-health-forum/fullarticle/2802872
11. MGMA. https://www.mgma.com/mgma-stats/healing-moral-injury-what-should-your-strategy-to-reduce-physician-burnout-look-like-

12. Physicians Foundation. https://physiciansfoundation.org/wp-content/uploads/PF23_Brochure-Report_Americas-Physicians_V2b-1-2.pdf
13. MGMA. https://www.mgma.com/mgma-stat/staying-vigilant-against-physician-burnout
14. JPS. https://www.jacksonphysiciansearch.com/physician-recruitment-roi-calculator/
15. https://www.mgma.com/mgma-stat/medical-groups-productivity-still-struggling-in-2023-amid-staffing-shortages
16. Adam Grant. "Think Again: The Power of Knowing What You Don't Know." 2021
17. Jennifer Deal. "Retiring the Generation Gap: How Employees Young and Old Can Find Common Ground." 2006.
18. MGMA. https://www.mgma.com/mgma-stats/physician-shortages-forcing-medical-group-leaders-to-be-more-flexible-in-their-staffing-models
19. JPS. https://www.jacksonphysiciansearch.com/back-from-burnout-confronting-the-post-pandemic-physician-turnover-crisis-2022-survey-results/
20. Physicians Thrive. https://physiciansthrive.com/physician-compensation/report/
21. Fierce Healthcare. https://www.fiercehealthcare.com/providers/physician-pay-rose-modest-3-2023-here-are-specialties-saw-biggest-gains
22. MGMA. https://www.mgma.com/mgma-stats/as-compensation-competition-continues-medical-group-leaders-say-staff-turnover-not-easing-up-yet

Chapter 6

Financial Models and Revenue Cycle Management Functions

By: Jonathan Leer, CHFP, CMPE

6.1 Introduction

As many who work in the healthcare industry may appreciate, the current healthcare delivery structure in the United States is fascinatingly complex. It exists as a unique blend of many components of the four major international healthcare delivery system models, which range in a spectrum from single-payer, fully tax-funded health coverage to fully out-of-pocket patient-funded coverage. For example, the Beveridge Model used in the United Kingdom is a model by which the government provides healthcare coverage to its citizens and the care is funded fully by taxes. Whereas many countries like India and those in much of Africa don't have a standard care delivery model and require that many of those citizens pay for care out of pocket.[1]

It may not be surprising then that care delivery models and financial models for medical practices within the United States can also exist on this broad spectrum of care delivery. For a medical practice to ensure its success and financial solvency overall, a critical first step is to ensure that the practice's financial model is in alignment with the practice's care delivery model. Once alignment between those two components exists, then RCM and operational techniques can be applied to appropriately maximize the practice revenue. This chapter will explore the primary healthcare delivery and financial models along with the key functions within those models.

Exhibit 6.1 Major Healthcare Delivery Models

Model	Description	Applicable Countries
Beveridge	Government is the sole payor; funded by income taxes	United Kingdom, Spain
Bismarck	Decentralized; mainly employee/employer funded	Germany, Japan, Switzerland
National Health Insurance	Blend of Beveridge and Bismarck; government as single payer	Canada, South Korea, Taiwan
Out-of-Pocket	Patient funded	India, China, Africa

6.2 Care Delivery & Financial Models

As healthcare resources have expanded and the population has grown in the United States, the mechanisms for providing care and paying for that care have become more complex. While America was once the land of simple fee-for-service coverage provided by independent physicians, clinics and hospitals, the advent of healthcare insurance, more complex healthcare organizations and the role of federal programs including Medicare, Medicaid and the Affordable Care Act coverage have produced a wider range of alternatives to both care delivery and financial responsibility.[2]

According to the AHA, the past decade has seen a significant shift as payers have increasingly moved a larger and larger portion of their payments for refined care delivery models, often referred to as alternative payment models or value-based payment models.[3] These work to incentivize providers for the quality and value of the care provided, versus pure volume of patients treated, as well as providing better healthcare outcomes. Alternative payment models also shift the financial risk to providers, so managers, administrators and physician owners are carefully watching as the changes occur. As the Healthcare Financial Management Association notes, "a forward-thinking financial model can help hospital

Chapter 6: Financial Models and Revenue Cycle Management Functions

leaders better predict and balance potential gains and losses from incentives, penalties, volume changes and other factors related to value-based payment."[4]

The Traditional Model: Fee for Service

Many healthcare management professionals are familiar with the United States' traditional and dominant payment model—the Fee-For-Service (FFS) model. This model has been in place for centuries and is built upon the premise that healthcare providers will bill separate fees to patients and/or their insurers for each service provided to a patient on a particular date of service.[5] What is particularly attractive about fee-for-service models is that they are predictable, as only services with an associated procedure code outlined in the Current Procedural Terminology (CPT) framework maintained by the American Medical Association (AMA) can be billed.[6] Currently many United States payors and medical groups leverage FFS billing in some way.

Some of the criticisms of the FFS model mention that this model is attributed to rising healthcare costs because it fundamentally rewards health providers to bill for the number of services rather than the quality of services provided, also it has not been proven to advance the improvement of health outcomes.[7] Additionally, from an operational and overhead perspective, FFS models require a significant amount of administrative and billing support to manage all the components required of the fee-for-service model, which can include contract negotiators, coders and financial personnel to manage patient payments.

A Newer Model: Value-Based Care

In an effort to enhance the FFS model, reduce healthcare costs and improve patient health outcomes, the Centers for Medicare and Medicaid Services (CMS) has begun to embark on establishing value-based care models through which "reimbursements are [in part] calculated by using numerous quality measures and determining the overall health of populations."[8] These include notions such as Accountable Care Organizations, Bundled Payments and Patient-Centered Medical Homes, as well as Provider-Sponsored Health Plans.[9] Through this construct of value-based care, medical providers and organizations are influenced to try to create efficiencies and use data-based methods for achieving metric goals. Specifically, in addition to billing FFS charges, healthcare providers are often assessed an incentive or penalty payment for achieving or failing to achieve the prescribed metrics of the program.

Value-based care is gaining interest, as over 25% of all FFS payments have had some linkage to quality and value as of 2020.[10] While the intent to reward medical providers for reducing costs and improving outcomes is noble, one such criticism of value-based care programs is that it is difficult for them to be universally applied across all practices and specialties. Therefore, they often have disparate or competing metrics which sometimes fail to align when overlaid with other programs. Additionally, many of these value-based programs are subject to medical providers opting in to participate and require that there be significant data-sharing across the practice and the program.

A Refreshed Model: Population-Based Payments

Although the population-based or capitated payments model is more dated than some of the newer value-based care models, this model is being refreshed from the original version that emerged in the 1980s. Through the reinvigorated capitated payments approach, providers receive a risk-adjusted, per-person payment that would cover that patient's prospective healthcare services over a prescribed time horizon.[11] Said in another way, this payment method tries to estimate healthcare payments across the responsible hospital or group's entire patient population for a specified time period, while adjusting for complex medical conditions to make one payment for the population's estimated total cost of care (TCC).

The goal of capitated payments is to incentivize care providers to help reduce waste (like ordering duplicate or unnecessary services or having to negotiate individual claims) while helping to reinforce providing quality care to a broad population. This model discourages billing based on the volume of services and establishes a goal for how much a care provider should expect to bill for one patient. One of the major benefits of capitation is that savings from waste elimination can be reinvested in the

Chapter 6: Financial Models and Revenue Cycle Management Functions

care delivery group to continue to foster an environment that improves health outcomes; however, capitation may not be a sustainable model for all practices and is one that passes a decent amount of the financial risk to the care provider.[12]

The Disruptor Model: Private Pay and Concierge

Considerably different and less egalitarian than other models, the model of concierge medicine has been around since the 1990s and seeks to simplify payments by assessing one fee (usually on a monthly or annual basis) in return for enhanced services like rapidly available appointment and communication response times. In this way, practices limit their patient population in most cases to just those who opt into that fee structure. In addition to removing the hassle and labor expense required of the medical insurance contracting and claims process, the benefits of this model include reducing administrative overhead, reducing the size of patient panels and increasing the quality of care provided per patient.[13] It is not without its drawbacks, as this model leaves behind most patients who cannot afford high out-of-pocket costs—so much so that some have challenged that this model carries with it a fundamental inequality related to income and wealth. It is also a model that is more common in primary care and less common in specialty and emergency care, so those who pay for concierge services may also still need to maintain health insurance for other required medical services.

Partnership Model: Independent Medical Practices and Larger Hospitals

While some might argue that the partnership model is not a care delivery or payment model per se, it is prudent to mention the importance and impact of hospital and medical practice alignments and partnerships on financial models. In an increasingly competitive U.S. healthcare environment, it is common for larger institutions to partner with community or private medical practices. The benefits of this partnership can be quite substantial and include increased regulatory adherence, improved negotiated contract rates, reductions in hospital and emergency department utilization rates, and increased data sharing and care coordination.[14]

Additionally, hospital-owned practices can leverage supporting infrastructure and can better integrate billing, medical records and other common administrative functions, which could provide economies of scale across a broader number of practices or medical groups.[15] One downside to this type of cooperative partnership is that sometimes it results in redundancies across a larger system and can be subject to higher charges passed onto patients. Hospital-regulated practices bill hospital fees in addition to the provider medical fees, and these hospital fees are not always covered by medical insurance leading to higher out-of-pocket or aggregate costs than a physician office bill.

Negotiating the changes in these evolving care delivery and financial payment structures will require healthcare managers and decision-makers to weigh the best mixture of patient care, financial simplicity and long-term risk management. The continued role of government payers will also continue to place more pressure on value-based care strategies.

6.3 Functions Within Care Delivery Models

While the traditional fee-for-service model established simple guidelines for payment responsibility and the internal mechanisms required to track and trace billable items, newer, more heavily government-funded or complex alternative models make it necessary to clearly outline the specific functions of the entire healthcare organization. Although not an exhaustive review, now that some of the common United States care and financial models have been discussed, it would be helpful to overview important revenue cycle management functions that help support the funds flow related to these models.

Revenue Cycle Management (RCM)

RCM can be defined as the integration of activities that support a patient visit encounter and end in some sort of revenue flowing into the practice. These activities can include:[16]

- Contracting
- Pre-visit activities
- Registration activities

Chapter 6: Financial Models and Revenue Cycle Management Functions

- Chart documentation
- Claims production
- Denial management
- Receivables management
- Post-audit and process improvement

Each of these RCM components plays a critical role in the overall integration of the revenue cycle and therefore each warrants its own overview.

Contracting (a.k.a. Managed Care Contracting)

Outside of the Concierge Model, most of the care delivery models—and especially the FFS model—operate with the understanding that there will be some sort of contractual agreement between the servicing medical provider and the payors, which can span either federal (e.g. Medicare/Medicaid) or private (e.g. Blue Cross Blue Shield) insurers. As a simplified example of contracting, a medical practice or provider can contract with an insurer with the intention to receive a fixed percentage of the cost of a service for payment.

Most often contract negotiations are guided by the CPT standardized coding framework, which ensures that there is a common definition, code and contracted payment for each associated procedure which allows all of the parties involved in the revenue cycle process to "speak the same language."[17] Due to the number and variety of insurers and payers, contracting can be a time-intensive process; however, some of the benefits of successful contracting include reduced administrative burdens for processing claims for services, improved revenue forecasting based on contractual arrangements and increased ability to treat a broader subset of patients.[18]

Pre-visit Activities

In all versions of the care delivery models, pre-visit activities are among some of the most important activities because they set the foundation for the patient encounter and how appropriate patient demographic and billing data are collected for use later in the cycle. Pre-visit activities can include patient scheduling, collecting pertinent patient identifying

125

information, verifying that the patient has insurance coverage and completing a benefit verification to determine which services may or may not be considered "covered" (or reimbursable) by the payor or contracted insurance agency.

Pre-visit activities can also include financial clearance and counseling, which ensure that the patient is aware of the potential charges and agrees to be billed for services that are not reimbursable by the insurance plan. While this component applies to the FFS structures, the same would hold with the concierge plans in that verification of annual fees paid would be required.

Registration Activities

During registration, the practice can ensure that the patient's pre-visit information is correct, which is not only important for FFS models but also important for the sharing of patient information for other models. For example, in the capitated payments and value-based care models, some of the metrics requirements and risk adjustments are made based on the patient's zip code or service area. So, collecting that information is just as important as collecting insurance information for the FFS plans. Another vital component of the registration activity is collecting any necessary co-pays or co-insurance in advance of the visit or procedure, which helps to reduce bad-debt collections, increase accounts receivables and help to maintain positive cash flow to the practice upstream from some of the latter parts of RCM.

Charting

At or around the time that care is delivered, there is usually a record of the services provided which is commonly referred to as charting. It is important for care providers to document all relevant information about the patient's encounter within the chart. For FFS models in the outpatient practice setting which are often billed by an evaluation & management (E/M) CPT code, there are dual methodologies for billing which include either quantifying the time that is required of a patient encounter or medical decision-making (MDM).[19] When charting based on time, it is important to note how much time was spent on the encounter, which

Chapter 6: Financial Models and Revenue Cycle Management Functions

can include both face-to-face and non-face-to-face time of the billing provider. When billing according to MDM, it is important for the provider to outline the extent of the patient's health problems and the extent of supporting data that needs to be reviewed and analyzed by the provider.[20]

Specifically, time-based billing can include things like review of prior tests and medical records, ordering medications and procedures and documenting clinical information on the date of the encounter, while MDM includes things like the complexity and number of the patient's medical problems and whether the provider needed to interpret tests independently or discuss those medical data with other specialists.[21] It becomes increasingly important for the provider or care teams to document things like complex medical problems for the value-based and capitated models since those data may need to be captured for assessing or quantifying metrics of the program or overall health of the patient population.

Claims Processing

Claims processing begins at the time a charge is "entered" for the patient encounter and the documentation is complete. Often for practices with electronic medical records (EMR) systems, the EMR system moves the bill to a common location (or workqueue) for the claims processors to begin their work.[22] A first step is usually to ensure that the documentation in the encounter note supports the CPT that was selected for billing by the care provider. If that criterion is not met, the processors can ask providers to addend the note or appropriately re-code the visit. Once the claim has been finalized, it is usually sent to the patient's insurance payor for payment, or the patient themselves in the event of self-pay patients. Since many payors have contractual requirements for timely claims processing, it is important to ensure that the documentation is completed and the claim is sent to the insurer within that established period.

Denial Management

The linkage between charting, claims production and claims denials is quite significant because appropriate documentation is a critical element that supports patient billing, irrespective of whether the encounter is billed via MDM or time. If the documentation is not adequate to support a billed service, that service may be denied or left unpaid by an insurer/payor. For example, a provider can bill a new patient consultation code based on the complexity of MDM, but in the absence of appropriate documentation for that code, the insurance can deny payment of the entire charge.

Even with the best intentions and documentation, it is still likely that a practice will experience a claim denial, which is a payor's refusal to pay for a billed service for a particular reason. Claim denials happen for a myriad of reasons, including typographical errors related to the entry of the patient's demographic or insurance information, lack of prior authorization, missing or incorrect site of service (e.g. inpatient versus medical office) or the services being deemed medically unnecessary or inappropriate.[23] In the event of a claim denial, practices can resubmit an amended claim for non-medical denials or file appeals for payment for medically denied claims.

Payments and Receivables Management

Provided everything goes according to plan in the steps of the revenue management cycle, the anticipated outcome is receiving payment for services billed. This often requires an established receivables management process that can reconcile payments against claims sent to insurers. A strong receivables management process will also facilitate data collection to enable continuous reporting which can allow for timely follow-up and requests for processing delayed payments and/or remaining patient balances. Additionally, specific receivables management processes may exist in parallel for those who participate in the capitated payments or value-based care models, and these processes may require an ability to reconcile how the data were reported, measured, and translated for payments.

Understanding the various stages and roles in revenue cycle management is the first step in optimizing efficient payment flow. With more attention to pre-visit authorizations and the appropriate registration and charting paperwork and electronic file-keeping, the incidence of claim denials can be reduced.

Chapter 6: Financial Models and Revenue Cycle Management Functions

Post Audit and Process Improvement

Just as important as the other RCM components, it is important to ensure that practices allocate time to consistent evaluation of the RCM process to identify components of the process that may be broken or could be improved to increase the cycle's efficiency. More specifically, collecting data on claims denial trends can help uncover whether improvements are needed in demographic data collection and whether charting is accurate if there is a high percentage of denials surrounding these two activities.

6.4 Key Performance Indicators

There are several metrics, also referred to as Key Performance Indicators (KPIs), which can measure the health of the practice's financial and RCM performance with some of the most prevalent outlined below. Measuring items before the visit, such as schedule utilization and financial clearance, can make claims processing and denial management an easier task. Close attention to metrics related to receivables management will also demonstrate the success (or shortcomings) of the entire RCM system.

Exhibit 6.2 Key Performance Indicators for RCM

RCM Component	Metric	Definition	Recommended Benchmark
Pre-visit Activities	Schedule utilization	Percentage of provider schedule utilized with scheduled appointments	100%+
	Financial Clearance	Percentage of patients who have been cleared by their appropriate insurance company for procedures/special appts.	98%
Claims Processing	Charge Lag	The number of days it takes from the encounter date to posting/sending the charge	<7 days
	Erroneous (or "clean") claim rate	The number of error-free claims over the total number of billed claims	>95%

RCM Component	Metric	Definition	Recommended Benchmark
Denial Management	Denial Rate	Percentage of payor claim denials over total submitted claims	No more than 2-3% of claims denied
	Denial Overturn	The number of denials subsequently approved over the total number of denials	>95%
Receivables Management	Days in accounts receivable	The average time it takes to receive payment for billed services	<30 days
	Bad debt expense	Percentage of net revenue that must be "written off" for non-payment	2-5% of Net Patient Revenue
	Gross collection ratio	The total cash received for a claim over the gross number of fees billed for the claim	>40-50%

It should be noted that those recommendations listed above are based upon our history in managing clinics over the years and do align with the organization where we currently are employed. These recommendations might vary based upon the size and the location of your clinic and its ownership structure. There are many KPIs that can be recommended and we would encourage reviewing MGMA's own website and education forums for up-to-date information about certain recommendations that relate to members across the association.

6.5 Practice in Action

A major independent provider of outpatient behavioral services found it difficult to get paid for services provided, and faced a mounting backlog due to its in-house and national accounts receivable (A/R) teams.[24] Revenue cycle KPIs demonstrated the problems: days in A/R topped out at 52 and the total outstanding 120-day A/R was nearly 30%, while the success of eligibility verifications was less than 80%.

Faced with financial threats to the entire organization, an outside consultant was enlisted to transform the existing RCM. New steps were instituted, which included a thorough denials analysis and identification of root causes, as well as a new eligibility verification process, with specialized insurance verification and denials management staff allocated to those roles. Clinicians and RCM leaders were also given more education to avoid denials, and a feedback loop was created for the front-end team to prevent denials, with more education on coding standards and insurance guidelines. Workflows were also structured to allow follow-up 21 days after each claim submission date.

The RCM metrics immediately demonstrated a significant change. Billing backlog was reduced from over 8 days to 0-1 days, and the total days in A/R were reduced from 52 days to 38 days. Claims 120-plus days in A/R also decreased from 28% to 15%, and the eligibility success rate improved from 80% to 94%. There was also a 4% increase in revenue per encounter and overall monthly collections increased from $5.1 million to $5.4 million.

6.6 Summary

The U.S. healthcare landscape is a complex ecosystem that consists of a blend of an infinite number of care delivery and financial models. Practices and practice managers need to understand the workings of each, and also the functions and pacing of the entire revenue cycle management system.

- Care delivery models have advanced from fee-for-service to value-based care models, with more oversight from the CMS. Other payment alternatives include population-based payments, private pay and concierge services, as well as partnerships between independent medical practices and larger hospitals.
- Revenue cycle management (RCM) includes the coordination of a range of activities such as contracting, pre-visit and registration activities, chart documentation, claims production and denial and receivables management.
- KPIs can be used to measure the success and performance of a practice's RCM procedures. Tracking pre-visit activities

such as financial clearance, plus claims processing and both denial and receivables management, can produce hard numbers on RCM objectives.

In the next chapter, we will look at the dynamics of payer contracting, and the best strategies for establishing financially expeditious relationships with payers through research, regular reviews and audits, as well as effective negotiation.

Notes

1. https://pphr.princeton.edu/2017/12/02/unhealthy-health-care-a-cursory-overview-of-major-health-care-systems/
2. AHA. https://www.aha.org/system/files/media/file/2019/04/MarketInsights_CareModelsReport.pdf
3. AHA. https://trustees.aha.org/aligning-care-delivery-emerging-payment-models
4. HFMA. https://www.hfma.org/payment-reimbursement-and-managed-care/value-based-payment/61962/
5. Bloomberg Law https://news.bloomberglaw.com/health-law-and-business/insight-the-healthcare-industrys-shift-from-fee-for-service-to-value-based-reimbursement
6. AMA. https://www.ama-assn.org/amaone/cpt-current-procedural-terminology
7. Dowd BE, Laugesen MJ. Fee-for-service payment is not the (main) problem . Health Services Research. 2020;55(4):491–5
8. https://revcycleintelligence.com/features/what-is-value-based-care-what-it-means-for-providers
9. AHA. https://trustees.aha.org/aligning-care-delivery-emerging-payment-models
10. Erickson SM, Outland B, Joy S, Rockwern B, Serchen J, Mire RD, et al. Envisioning a better U.S. Health Care System for all: Health Care Delivery and payment system reforms. Annals of Internal Medicine. 2020;172
11. HBR https://hbr.org/2016/07/the-case-for-capitation
12. Cox T. Exposing the true risks of capitation financed healthcare. Journal of Healthcare Risk Management. 2011 Jan. 30 (4):34–41.
13. NLMhttps://pubmed.ncbi.nlm.nih.gov/27892907/
14. Lockett KM. Integrating hospital and physician revenue cycle operations. Healthcare Finance Manage. 2014 Mar;68(3)
15. Hilts KE, Yeager VA, Gibson PJ, Halverson PK, Blackburn J, Menachemi N. Hospital Partnerships for Population Health: A systematic review of the literature. Journal of Healthcare Management. 2022Jan1;66(3):170–98.

Chapter 6: Financial Models and Revenue Cycle Management Functions

16. Mugdh M, Pilla S. Revenue cycle optimization in Health Care Institutions. The Health Care Manager. 2012;31(1):75–80.
17. Dotson P. CPT® codes: What are they, why are they necessary, and how are they developed? Advances in Wound Care. 2013Oct9;2(10):583–7.
18. Ly DP, Glied SA. The impact of managed care contracting on physicians. Journal of General Internal Medicine. 2013Sep4;29(1):237–42.
19. AMA. https://www.ama-assn.org/topics/evaluation-and-management-em-coding
20. NIH. https://www.ncbi.nlm.nih.gov/pmc/articles/PMC9560052/
21. AMA https://www.ama-assn.org/system/files/2019-06/cpt-office-prolonged-svs-code-changes.pdf
22. HFMA. https://www.hfma.org/technology/revenue-cycle-technology/how-healthcare-organizations-navigate-claims-processing/
23. https://www.medicaleconomics.com/view/improve-claims-management-process-preventing-payer-denials
24. Access Healthcare. https://www.accesshealthcare.com/case-study/efficient-accounts-recovery-delivers-impressive

Chapter 7

Payer Contracting

By: Doral Jacobsen, MBA, FACMPE

7.1 Introduction

This chapter will provide insights regarding payer contracting for medical practices to consider and share the approaches of better performing practices. It all starts with appreciating that payer contracting is a foundational part of the revenue cycle, as each payer represents a contribution to the bottom line. Payers build networks to contract with practices or other aggregators—e.g., Independent Practice Associations (IPAs) or Clinically Integrated Networks—and must create a network that can support their customers.

According to the AMA, a payer is "an entity that pays for services rendered by a healthcare provider."[1] Payers can range from individual patients to employers, government payers and commercial insurance companies. Other contracted payers can also include third-party administrators or other intermediate entities. As the AMA's Payer Contracting 101 explains, "The identity of a payer may determine the degree to which terms are fixed or negotiable, the applicable laws, negotiating strategy and goals and objectives of the relationship."

Payer contracting is a key focus area for medical practices that is both extremely challenging to manage and is critically important. Practices are responsible for routinely requesting increases to existing rates to ensure escalating costs are covered. Innovative payment models are being piloted and implemented in markets across the country and practices are pressed to consider new types of data and administrative burden associated with these contracts. New payers emerge constantly and practices must determine if participation is warranted. Payer claim edits continue to erode revenue and somehow fade into background as they negatively impact the bottom line.[2] Administrative burden is a constant challenge for practices which do not add value and are not routinely considered as part of the contract negotiation process. Finally, monitoring contract performance is rarely integrated with practice key performance indicators which often leads to the common situation of falling to the bottom of the priority list.

Dealing with those rate increases, coping with the issues related to adapt to new payment models, coping with new payers and more successfully integrating KPIs with contract performance are all key challenges. Medical practices are not always equipped with the skill sets and bandwidth to develop and deploy a successful payer contracting strategy. While it is a tough landscape to navigate, practices can set themselves up to thrive if they're armed with a solid framework and straightforward strategy.

Without practices, payers have nothing to offer employers/members. Payers can offer multiple product lines including but not limited to: Commercial, Medicare, Medicaid, Workers' Compensation, Automotive and others. Practices contract with payers either directly or indirectly and the first challenge is getting your arms around this universe. Of course government payers such as Medicare and Medicaid require monitoring and managing and in some cases negotiation as well. This chapter will also focus on negotiation strategies that are relevant across payers and will provide specific examples for all negotiable books of business.

7.2 Review Contract Performance

An August 2023 MGMA Stat Poll found that some 58% of medical groups review their payer contracts on an annual basis.[3] Contract terms often dictate when a medical practice should start the negotiation conversation, but other factors—such as legislative changes, market dynamics in

Chapter 7: Payer Contracting

healthcare, reimbursement rate changes, performance metrics and quality indicators—can drive the conversation for new contract terms.

Cataloging contracts is the first framework element necessary to deploy a successful payer contracting strategy. For each contractual relationship, better performing practices acquire the following:

- **Fully executed agreements and amendments:** Contract signed by the practice and the payer
- **Fee Schedules:** For each product the practice should understand exactly what is expected in terms of allowable for services and load this information into the billing system
- **Value-based program key elements:** Program criteria, reports from payer, reconciliation approach and payer meetings
- **Administrative Burden:** By payer, a running list of the administrative burdens that create work that does not add value (i.e., prior authorizations, incorrect payments)

Obtain executed agreements and fee schedule extracts from payers for all major contracts and make details available to the revenue cycle team.

A key challenge for administrators is gathering the feedback described above relative to contract performance—practices rarely have all of these pieces of the puzzle. Practices with advanced skills in this area have some common practices that focus on the end goal painting the picture of key elements necessary to evaluate contract performance annually. This approach empowers the revenue cycle team to become part of the payer contracting workflow and provide valuable insights for upcoming negotiations. Inviting the revenue cycle team to participate in the contracting cycle ensures that the approach is comprehensive and that pain points are understood and addressed. The revenue cycle team holds the key and if this is a contracted service this still holds true.

Below are advanced workflows of practices employ:

Quarterly: Review payer contracting Key Performance Indicators (KPIs) for major payers:

- **Payer Mix:** Total Charges for each payer
- **Gross Collections:** Payments divided by Charges
- **Reimbursement Accuracy:** Percentage of payments correctly paid
- **Billed Charge compared to allowables:** Determine highest rate for each CPT code and ensure that charges exceed the rate
- **Accounts Receivable (AR) Aging Buckets:** Percentage of AR over 90 days outstanding
- **Administrative Burden:** Running list of billing team pain points
- **Denials:** Categorized by payer in terms of percentage of payments by payer
- **Aggregate Percentage of Medicare:** In terms of current year what the practice is paid based on contracted rates compared to Medicare rates
- **Value-based revenue:** Dollars attributed to value-based contract elements
- **Negotiation Status:** Last negotiation conclusion date and outcome, next negotiate target date and necessary preparation steps

Schedule a connection call with major payers (30 minutes include agenda and take minutes), then integrate executive summary of payer contracting performance into strategy reported to owners.

Monthly: Complete a Revenue Cycle Team Meeting and gather/discuss KPI collection including trends, report on payer website updates to identify policy changes that may impact the practice.

Integrate payer contracting as part of RCM and provide business owners with regular updates regarding contract performance and strategy status.

This is a robust approach and much like other efforts (e.g., standing up a telehealth platform) once in place it becomes part of the standard workflow. The benefits are enormous in that practices able to get arms around this data and normalize communication routines have a deep understanding of the value of each relationship. Also, this approach engages practice resources that have critical knowledge and allows the practice to leverage this information in negotiations.

For example, revenue cycle team members understand how much time is wasted on pre-payment audits, clinicians have a view into cost savings based on site of service etc. Payer contracting status in turn informs overall practice strategy and assists in determining which payer relationships are working well and which ones are in need of improvement or retirement. It also provides key questions practices can use in assessing new relationships to ensure that it will be a good fit for the organization. Creating this framework will allow practice executives to pull together a comprehensive picture of payer contracts and enable effective prioritization annually. According to a January 2021 MGMA Stat Poll, 47% of healthcare leaders audit their payer contracted rates on an annual basis, which can help evaluate the effectiveness and reliability of all clinical documentation in health records and billing data submitted to payers.[4]

7.3 Compare Contract Performance

Once the key catalog elements and KPIs described previously have been obtained, practices can assess contract performance based on the following high level criteria: fee for service rates, value-based revenue or penalty, and administrative burden cost to the practice.[5] According to Enter, a revenue cycle management provider, these considerations should be evaluated for all major payers, as they drive 3-5% or more revenue annually and compared across payers considering renegotiation windows.[6] This information is utilized to define payer targets for renegotiation on an ongoing basis. Primary targets include major payer contracts that are within the negotiation window, meaning that the term of the last contract has expired and the rates/model are in need of incremental increase due to inflation, administrative burden or payment model considerations. Payers that drive less revenue to the practice should also be evaluated and prioritized as necessary.

For example, if administrative burden is significant but the payer drives low volume to the practice, the relationship should be evaluated to determine if discussion is warranted to reduce the burden. If the payer is unwilling to accommodate, the practice can consider exiting the arrangement. Also, small payers are in prime position to capture market share, which happens frequently. Smaller payer fee schedules are usually low as practices drop negotiations to the bottom of the list and the repercussions can be very disadvantageous. According to accounting and consulting firm Weaver, a stable payer mix is crucial to premium valuation.[7] Consider what happens when a large state employer moves from a large payer to a more obscure one overnight. Such a transition can have a significant financial impact.

Also consider aggregate fee for service percentage of Medicare, administrative burden, payer mix, negotiation target dates and value-based impact when creating an annual payer contracting strategy and prioritize payers considering the potential overall impact to practice bottom line.

Comparing contract performance across payers provides the framework for strategy development. The information collected can be boiled down to three key considerations: last increase to overall rates, administrative burden and economic impact of potential rate negotiation. Advanced strategies include this comprehensive analysis:

Exhibit 7.1 Payer Contract Performance Analysis

Payer	Years – Last Increase	Admin Burden	Estimated Economic Impact	Total
Payer 1	5	5	5	15
Payer 2	1	3	3	7
Payer 3	4	5	5	14
Payer 4	1	3	3	7
Payer 5	2	3	2	7
1 – low	2 – low/medium	3 – medium	4 – medium/high	5 – highest

The last increase score considers when the contract received a rate increase either through fee for service lift or value-based methodology or a combination of both. Contracts that have not been negotiated in recent years become a priority focus. Administrative burden ranking considers denials, billing team pain points, AR aging and reimbursement accuracy. The higher the score the more taxing the payer indicating that it costs the practice more to be contracted with the payer and this consideration should be included in the negotiation. The estimated economic impact evaluates volume in terms of payer mix/revenue, aggregate percentage of Medicare and gross collections. Payers that rank high on potential return are prioritized. The chart below depicts the analyses:

Exhibit 7.2 Payer Contract Comparison

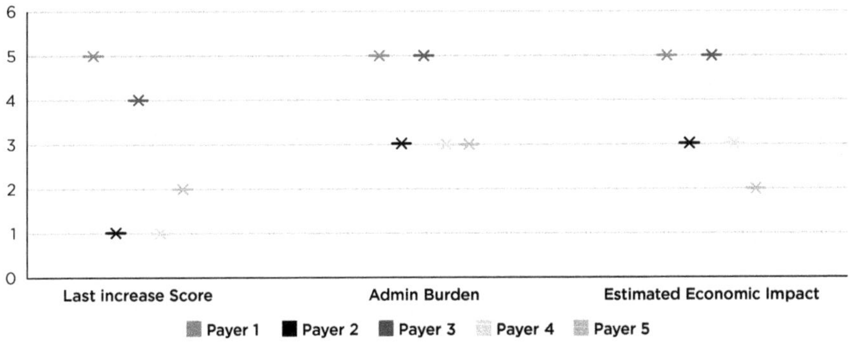

Based on this analysis, Payers 1 and 3 would be prioritized as primary targets with Payers 2 and 4 as secondary targets. Payer 5 would be monitored and focused on if possible but only after primary and secondary target negotiations are well underway. This type of analysis brings the key considerations together and supports executives in communicating payer contracting strategy by focusing on the most critical payers in an understandable prioritization order.

7.4 Define Payer Targets and Proposals

Once payers targets have been identified for the year, the practice turns to developing proposals for each payer of interest. Proposals are developed considering the following elements:

- Fee for service rates
- Last negotiation date
- Last increase % and cost to provide services
- Administrative burden score
- APM impact (economic/administrative burden)
- Products of interest
- New service offerings
- Market considerations
- Practice contracting affiliations

In terms of fee for service rates, better performers calculate a baseline for each contract based on current year Medicare. As every payer utilizes different methodology to establish contract rates, a normalized weighted average analysis is necessary to determine the relative value of the contract to the practice. Below is a depiction of the analysis which will provide a fee for service aggregate equivalency which in the example is 107% of Medicare.

Exhibit 7.3 Fee for Service Aggregate Equivalency

CPT	Description	Contracted Rate Payer A	Medicare	%Mcare	Total Volume	Est Total Payment = Rate*Vol	Est Total Medicare Payment = Mcare * Vol
99213	Office Visit	$75	$70	107%	5,000	$375.000	$350.000
69210	Ear Wax Removal	$65	$50	130%	500	$32.500	$25.000
90471	Immunization admin	$20	$25	80%	500	$10.000	$12.500
83036	Glycosylated hemoglobin test	$8	$15	53%	500	$4.000	$7.500
Totals						$421,500	$395,000
Fee for Service Aggregate Equivalency						107%	

Once this analysis has been completed for payer targets, fee for service aggregate equivalency can be compared across payers, as in this sample chart.

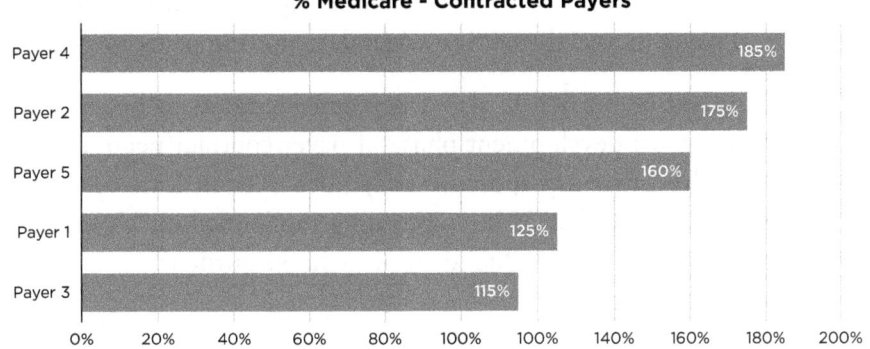

Exhibit 7.4 Medicare Contracted Payers Sample Chart

% Medicare - Contracted Payers

Payer	%
Payer 4	185%
Payer 2	175%
Payer 5	160%
Payer 1	125%
Payer 3	115%

Payers 1 and 3 are lower in this comparison which impacts the potential economic impact of a negotiation. There is more ground to make up with these payers and this type of comparison clarifies the potential for contracts considering practice contracts.

Better performing practices constantly negotiate payer contracts. Payers provide the practice "paycheck" and in effect, when practices do not prioritize contract negotiations they are pressed to cover ever increasing costs without additional dollars. Of course, this is the situation to be avoided and negotiations for major payers are recommended annually or every other year. Understand that payers budget for increases anticipated in the network and by negotiating and obtaining increases your practice essentially enters the payer budget, which is the goal.

As payers increase premiums to cover cost of care, increasing administrative costs to the provider should be anticipated as well. Practices can access payer financial data, which is commonly available through the state department of insurance. The rate filing contains trend information which can be useful in negotiations. Additionally, a medical consumer price index (MCPI) is available through the U.S. Bureau of Labor Statistics, which covers services that are performed and billed by private-practice medical doctors, dentists, eye care providers and other medical providers.[8] Practices can compare rates for most common services provided compared to cost to provide the service/supply and leverage this data in negotiations as well.

In addition to the timeline of the last increase from payers, consider inflationary costs relative to MCPI, practice expenses, cost to provide services and payer financial trending when determining payer proposals.

Administrative burden is also a key consideration to be assessed during the proposal development phase of payer contract negotiations. Appreciating that currently approximately 30% of healthcare spending is considered waste, of that 30%—according to Council on Healthcare Spending and Value—half is due to administrative burden.[9]

Practices can assess and articulate these burdens as part of negotiations to provide a fuller picture of the economic impact of burdens driven by payer protocols. The revenue cycle team has this information and, as part of proposal preparation, better performers clearly articulate issues and desired resolutions for payers to consider as part of the negation process. For example, the list below is a high level sample list of issues/resolutions:

Exhibit 7.5 Payer Negotiation Issues/Resolutions

Payer 1 Admin Burden Issue	Desired Outcome
Pre-payment audits	Remove practice from pre-payment audits
Prior authorization requirements	Green Light practice for prior authorizations
Risk Adjustment Audits	Charge per chart $$$$ and limit request to no more than XX per year.

Be prepared to describe scenarios and also have examples for discussion to ensure that this information can be easily provided to payers if necessary.

Alternative payment model impact should be assessed as well in proposal preparation. Models may incorporate bonus programs and/or share risks elements. The practice should consider if the program is producing projected outcomes in terms of estimated economic impact in relationship to practice performance. In some cases, practices forgo fee for service increases in lieu of bonus programs and the overall impact should be evaluated to determine if the model is producing desired results for all involved.

Perform mid-year evaluation of performance in APM contract methodologies to determine if estimated performance is on target and meet with payer partners to review findings.

Proposal Preparation

Part of proposal preparation includes assessing payer product options as well as practice growth strategy relative to new service offerings. According to the Healthcare Financial Management Association, this requires supporting all contract proposals and requests with accurate data and analytics.[10] A review of available products should be completed as can be accomplished by reviewing payer websites, asking payer contracting representatives for the list of current available products and also inquiring with the revenue cycle team regarding this potential pain point. Compare results with the current contract product participation list and determine if practice requests should include adding or subtracting products. If the payer has denied participation with a narrow network, add this to the meeting agenda. At times, payers base decisions on narrow network participation on provide categorization that can be incorrect.

Explore this decision with payers as we see that many times this can be resolved if incorrect data assumptions are at the root of the issue. Also, consider future service offerings and compare contracts to understand potential impact to reimbursement rates and/or APM programs. Consider the default methodology and assess implications as part of proposal creation. For example, if the payer contract defaults to a "market schedule" for new services not provided by Medicare, consider requesting a default at a percentage of billed charges.

Overall market and practice affiliation considerations also need to be assessed in preparation for negotiations. Some questions to pose include the following:

Market Share

- What is the practice market share compared to last year?
- What is the payer market share compared to last year?
- What are potential future considerations?

Competitors

- How many competitors in the network this year compared to last year?
- What are volumes in terms of service provided this year compared to last?

Contracting Vehicles

- What contracting options are available for this payer contract?
- What is the cost of contracting vehicles?

Compile findings for each payer target and establish the practice proposal. The chart below depicts a working compilation that can be referenced as the proposal is drafted for payer considerations. It is also advisable to create a negotiation timeline and back into tasks to accomplish each milestone as the practice moves through negotiations.

Exhibit 7.6 Payer Consideration Sample

Contract Consideration	Payer 1
Fee for service rates	Current 125% Medicare
Last negotiation date	4 Years ago
Last increase %	3%
Administrative burden score	D
APM impact (economic / administrative burden)	Penalty -1%
Products of interest	Exchange product new request to add to contract
New service offerings	Adding infusion services next year—request rates / add to contract
Market considerations	20% of payer mix, volume same as last year practice / payer market share
Practice contracting affiliations	IPA contract available but this payer not option
Proposal	175% of Medicare over two years and remove value-based program if not revised, resolve prepayment audit burden and add exchange product to contract as well as infusion services

Each payer contract should be considered and the last quarter of the year is an ideal time to craft a strategy for the next year—be it calendar or fiscal. Establish a contracting timeline and commit the resources—either outsource or internal—to deploy the strategy on an ongoing basis.

7.5 Deploy Negotiation Communication Plan

In terms of overall communication plans, there are a few foundational elements to consider. The first thing to consider is developing a value proposition that frames the practice's value for discussion. Then there are communication pathways to consider which include in person meetings, virtual meetings, phone calls, letters and emails. The value proposition is essential and is really an enjoyable component of negotiations. Creating this content will assist the practice in recognizing and quantifying the value the practice brings to the healthcare ecosystem. Communicating the initial proposal and assessing when to utilize other methods as negotiations proceed is critical to the process. Pulling this plan together will assist executing a successful negotiation communication plan and create historical references for future negotiations.

Value Proposition

The value proposition is the document that will be circulated internally at the payer.[11] The goal of the value proposition is to tell your practice story and gain an advocate at the payer. The contracting representative has a range of increase that can be provided to the practice, and if the practice request is higher than what they can provide the proposal will be escalated internally. The value proposition can ride alongside the request which supports the proposal. This saves time and also minimizes the potential implications of the "telephone game" where once the message passes through a few people it does not even remotely resemble the actual facts.

A practice value proposition contains the following information:

Market Position

- Clinicians in terms of number, type and specialty
- Services provided

- Locations
- Accreditations, certifications
- Accolades

Value

- Mission statement
- Ratings by payers and other entities (e.g., vitals, google)
- Patient testimonials
- Quality programs with results compared to benchmarks / peers
- Cost efficiency with estimates of savings

Collaboration

- Healthcare Effectiveness Data and Information Set (HEDIS) Measures that are specific to the payer of interest[12]
- Quadruple Aim establishing overall goals
- Value program goals
- Questions / Next Steps

Create a comprehensive insightful value proposition that clearly explains the practice's benefit to the payer, quantifies cost savings and demonstrates a focus on quality care.

The value proposition can be crafted in written form or by using a more graphic approach such as PowerPoint or other graphic tools. It should be simple and easy to understand and adding visual components make it more interesting and eye catching. In terms of market position, this is the nuts and bolts of the practice. Many times payers are not aware of services provided, size of group, etc., and refreshing the conversation with this information provides key facts for the payer.

Many times certain payment models have thresholds for participation and including this data give the payer information needed to assess options for the group if this path is of interest. The value piece of the value proposition should anchor why the payer wants to keep the practice in the network. Highlighting quality programs aligns with what payers work on every day to boost ratings. Demonstrating how a practice bends the

Chapter 7: Payer Contracting

cost curve, such as providing access for patients as an alternative to an emergency room visit, also supports the request for increase.

Essentially, the practice is asking for a portion of savings created. The collaboration section is a more forward-facing position for new models and also connects the dots between HEDIS rates and how the practice helps the payer star ratings. New models can be financially rewarding and as collaboration opportunities are discussed, be sure to understand the administrative burden to make sure the juice is worth the squeeze.

Once the value proposition has been created, a communication plan typically follows the rhythm below:

The methods to communicate include emails, calls, virtual meetings, letters and in-person meetings. Emails are the most common—they are trackable and saving these is a best practice. Getting a payer by phone is a great way to build relationships and schedule the next follow-up touch point, saving a lot of back and forth. For phone interactions, be sure to follow up with a summary in writing specifying the next steps for all parties with due dates. Don't forget to use humor—this is a great way to build relationships and goes a long way with contracting reps as the day is usually filled with many unhappy practices. The recommendation is to be "180 degrees" in terms of approach from others, which will help the practice and the payer in the negotiation process immensely.

The best option is a face-to-face meeting as the opportunity to connect is substantially increased. The practice has an opportunity to share more about the practice such as providing a tour. For example, a multi-specialty group with a lab provided a payer with a tour of the lab and explained the quick turnaround time to the payer. Payers are notorious for low lab rates, and providing this context gives the practice an opportunity to demonstrate the value of the lab. It also visually shares the investment required to provide this level of service. These are the topics that get lost in translation. If you can get the payer in person the impact is greater. Another tactic that is useful is simply asking questions that get the payer to think about the practice's position from the provider perspective. For example, ask if they understand what expense increases the practice has experienced in the last few years or how many of their members have that practice cared for after normal business hours. This provides a more engaging launching pad for further discussion along with the quantification of practice value.

Once the practice has connected with the payer and provided value proposition information, send the proposal and establish a rhythm to follow up on the response. The proposal should include the increase of rates desired, specific administrative burden issues that require resolution and any value based considerations as well. This is typically sent via email and tenacious follow-up is the next phase of the process. A typical rhythm is every other week and best practices insert phone calls with the payer into the mix. Many times the verbal dialogue helps clear up questions and support moving the negotiation forward.

Pick up the phone during the negotiation process and focus on gaining an advocate to assist in moving the negotiation forward.

7.6 Evaluate Proposals/Counters

In terms of response to the practice's proposal, there are a few possibilities in terms of response to rates:

- No response
- Proposal denied
- Counter received from payer less than current rates
- Counter received from payer break-even
- Counter received from payer better than current rates but significantly less than from proposal
- Counter received from payer at or better than proposal

If the payer does not respond to the request or flat out denies the proposal, put in a phone call to the contract representative. Many times this gets the ball rolling and if they continue to be non-responsive, escalate to executives at the payer. Websites or search tools can be used to identify these individuals. Draft a letter to the payer requesting reconsideration and push for a meeting. Common targets for these communications include: Chief Executive Officer, Chief Medical Officer (CMO), and Vice Presidents of Contracting. Consider having clinicians sign these communications as this can carry more weight especially if the CMO from the payer side has been involved in the process.

If the response received is a break even, worse than current rates or far off from desired rates—keep pushing. This is the hard part and there are few options to consider:

- Counter with a lesser amount than initial proposal and spread the increase over multiple years
- Terminate the agreement, at time negotiations get a kick start with this method

Determine the practice's "walk away" point, be it a percentage of Medicare or targeted increase, and play out the scenarios. Examine the situation holistically, evaluating the cost of the contract to the practice in terms of administrative burden, cost to provide services, value-based program bonuses and how the payer fits into to overall strategy while considering market share goals in addition to fee for service rates. Deep dive and involve physicians in the discussion and look at it from a business perspective. It is ok to let the payer know that the practice is considering termination if that is possible, but be ready to pull the trigger if necessary. If termination is issued, many times payers come back to the table, but this is not guaranteed.

Evaluate the payer relationship holistically and if the contract does not align with practice values and overall strategy, address gaps during negotiations or exit the contract.

The last and amazingly best possible outcome is that the payer proposed more than requested—and yes this does happen. This is due at times to age of contract, methodology update on the payer side and make certain that the current and proposed rates are correct and move forward with language review.

7.7 Negotiate Language/Execute Agreement

Once rates have been agreed upon, the contract or amendment will need to be reviewed. The documents should be read completely while flagging any questions for the payer if clauses are unclear and/or concerning. According to Penny Noyes, CHC, president and CEO of Health Business Navigators, medical group practice leaders need to keep a sharp eye for unusual or obscure language when finalizing these agreements.[13] Noyes cautions administrators to be especially careful of phrases such as "joint construction," what constitutes the "lesser of" a particular contract rate, or language discussing termination rights or less favorable notice provisions.

We will cover the highlights in this section in order to establish minimum requirements for review and outline common potholes. Agreements and amendments should be reviewed at a minimum for the following:

- **Rates:** Are they clearly described and accurate by product?
- **Term:** How long will the practice be participating?
- **Termination:** How and when can the practice exit the agreement?
- **Penalties:** Are there any penalties and what could they mean to the practice financially?

Rates

Regarding rates, a best practice is to have the payer provide a fee extract in a format that can be uploaded into practice management software. If this is not provided, provide estimates and have the payer verify the rates. Be sure to fully read this section to understand if any exclusions apply to the practice and how each service, supply, vaccine etc. will be reimbursed. If certain categories will be adjusted, understand the timing. Also, review the products and ask if there are any products the practice will not be included in the agreement.

Term

Length of agreement should be reviewed to ensure that payers are not locking the practice into an arrangement for multiple years without escalating increases. For example, if the contract has a term of three years, request automatic increases in subsequent years to cover escalating costs. If the payer pushes back, take a look at their rate filing which may be available through the departments of insurance, which will describe premium increases. This is just the cost of doing business. Leverage by asserting that in order to be sustainable, inflationary costs must be considered and cite the rate filing. Also, utilize geographic inflation trends to substantiate the request, which is available through the Bureau of Labor Statistics.[14]

Termination

Perhaps the most critical clause is termination. How does the practice exit the contract? The best case is at any time with cause with relatively short notice (e.g., 60 or 90 days). Work to prevent being locked into an agreement for more than a year, especially if there are no escalators embedded on an annual basis. This can be a deal breaker for practices. Along these lines, understand how the payer can amend the contract and request dual signatures for all amendments that are not statutory requirements. Most contracts give the payer an out at any time for any reason, and requesting reciprocity here is reasonable.

Penalties

Penalties are embedded in many contracts and are found in many places. This is why it is important to peruse the contract in its entirety to identify these clauses and request removal. Be specific relative to the page(s) where they are found and if the clause is repeated be sure they remove all of the clauses. They can range from penalties for incorrect coding to decreases in fee schedules for defining time periods based on payer discretion.

In terms of communicating language requests, the best practice is to redline the agreement, which means adding comments to the document and moving through the process. If that is not possible, create a document and include the clause as written along with requested revisions and rationale for request. Submit the request to the payer and move through the process by reviewing the final document to make sure revisions have been completed as agreed. Many times payers do not update these documents accurately and the onus is ultimately on the practice to sign the correct versions. Once the contract has been completed, send it to the payer and follow up to obtain an effective date, then assign the next start date for renegotiation. End a contract negotiation by identifying the start date for the next renegotiation and keep renegotiating agreements on a routine basis.

7.8 Practice in Action

The negotiation process in payer contracting, like any other negotiation, requires you to tap into your behavior awareness of both yourself and those who you negotiate with. Many people are afraid to address uncomfortable topics and have few strategies in ensuring that discussions are impactful. I recently shared some of my personal payer contracting negotiation experience and tactics, during an MGMA Women in Healthcare podcast.[15]

We do so many things that fall in line with the whole "never split the difference" thought process, but one of the tactics that we use routinely is called tactical empathy. It's really listening to what is happening on the other side and aligning with it, because in contrast to a lot of our peer groups, we don't come out with guns blazing—we are very collaborative in our approach. Most of us are from the payer side, so we understand what it's like to sit in that seat. Aligning with the payer and trying to be a problem solver is where we come from. By being empathetic to the payer, we create connectivity, which is probably one the reasons why we're so successful with our clients. That connectivity helps us as a catalyst to launch into all kinds of things like discussions about innovative models or different scenarios that we might try out over time to solve problems for a practice.[16]

Another thing that I would say we use quite often is mirroring. When we're trying to get information from a payer, we always start our conversations by asking the payer a little bit about what's happening in their world, how long they've been there and what have been their roles, because folks like to talk about themselves. It's like a launching pad for finding out about new products and new initiatives. We use mirroring a lot so we can better understand what's going on with the payer and we can help the payer understand what the value is that the practice brings. That is helpful in terms of what their initiatives are.

However, don't be the person that emails the payer and says, "We need a 50% increase tomorrow." Really get in there, listen, be collaborative and make it easy for the payer to understand the value that your practice brings to the organization ,and quantify it. Every practice I talk to is a high-quality practice that asks itself, "what did the numbers show and how does that compare to benchmarks?" So looking at that information is going to help you position in a negotiation. Prioritizing it, putting it in the strategic plan and then rolling it out as a long term objective is going to help you make sure that you ask for those increases when you need to. A lot of these contracts have renewal windows, and if you miss them, they're in that contract for another year. So it's really important to get ahead of it.

7.9 Summary

Payer contracting is a cycle. It is iterative and evolves like other business functions in practices. However, it is not a highly visible workflow and most contracts are evergreen and continue forever, unless the practice takes a step to reflect on the contract and renegotiate for more favorable rates. Here are some of this chapter's highlights on those strategies:

- Conduct regular reviews of payer contract performance, on a monthly, quarterly and annual basis, to better understand agreements and amendments, fee schedules, value-based program elements and the overall administrative burden. Use payer contracting KPIs to benchmark those trends.
- Compare contract performance using fee for service rates and value-based revenues or penalties. Examine payers' last increase to their rates, their administrative burden and the economic impact of rate negotiation.
- Establish payer targets and proposals. Examine their market share, competitors and contracting vehicles.
- Deploy a negotiation communication plan. Create a well-researched value proposition statement, and then arrange both personal and electronic interactions to help build relationships.
- Evaluate the proposals and determine the counter proposals, in light of the practice's objectives.
- Negotiate the language and execute the agreement, if factors including rates, term, termination and penalties are acceptable.

In the next chapter, we will examine the uses of data in optimizing healthcare operations, including the value of benchmarking against other competitors. The vast variety of electronic records and financial statements generated by a healthcare organization yield a stream of data which can be used to help make better allocations of resources and staff.

Notes

1. AMA. https://www.ama-assn.org/system/files/payor-contracting-toolkit.pdf
2. 6Degrees Health. https://www.6degreeshealth.com/what-is-claim-editing-sdh/
3. https://www.mgma.com/mgma-stat/is-it-time-to-review-your-groups-payer-contracts
4. MGMA. https://www.mgma.com/mgma-stats/new-year-s-resolution-optimizing-audits-of-your-medical-practice-s-payer-contracted-rates
5. CMS. https://www.cms.gov/medicare/payment/fee-schedules
6. Enter. https://www.enter.health/post/healthcare-future-value-based-care-revenue-cycle-management
7. Weaver. https://weaver.com/resources/importance-stable-payer-mix-premium-valuation/
8. U.S. Bureau of Labor Statistics. https://www.bls.gov/cpi/factsheets/medical-care.htm
9. American College of Physicians. https://www.acponline.org/practice-resources/business-resources/payment/medicare-payment-and-regulations-resources/macra-and-the-quality-payment-program/alternative-payment-models-apms
10. HFMA. https://www.hfma.org/payment-reimbursement-and-managed-care/how-providers-can-optimize-payer-contract-negotiations/
11. CMS. https://www.cms.gov/priorities/innovation/files/x/tcpi-valuepropguide.pdf
12. Health.gov. https://health.gov/healthypeople/objectives-and-data/data-sources-and-methods/data-sources/healthcare-effectiveness-data-and-information-set-hedis
13. MGMA. https://www.mgma.com/articles/what-to-watch-for-when-negotiating-payer-contracts-in-2018
14. Bureau of Labor Statistics. https://www.bls.gov/
15. MGMA. https://www.mgma.com/podcasts/women-in-healthcare-healthcare-payer-contracting-and-personal-growth-insights-from-doral-jacobsen
16. Health Affairs. https://www.healthaffairs.org/do/10.1377/hpb20220909.830296/

Chapter 8

The Data Scene

By: David Gans,
MSHA, FACMPE

"One accurate measurement is worth a thousand expert opinions."

—Rear Admiral Grace Hopper (1906-1992)

8.1 Introduction

Increased costs due to inflation and investments in new technologies are affecting all healthcare organizations—but government and commercial insurer contracts are not increasing payment.

With higher costs and static payment, what can you do?

- Increase productivity to get more bang for the buck
- Reduce costs to get the same bang for less bucks
- Improve revenue cycle performance to get more bucks for the bang

In this chapter, we will learn that by comparing the data that a practice accumulates during its normal operations to national standards and to that of "better performing" practices, one can assess how each strategy will improve the bottom line and what is needed to do to remain viable and to thrive in an uncertain healthcare environment.

We will also take a close look at mining that data for key performance indicators (KPIs) and using them to set benchmarks against similar healthcare organizations that balance value and cost. It is important to identify both financial and non-financial metrics so you will have a comprehensive view of the practice. It is also important to structure your practice's electronic health record, billing and practice management information systems to aggregate data on an ongoing basis so you will have the KPIs you need for benchmarking success.

As the healthcare environment evolves, your practice needs to evolve as well. In the future, your organization needs the "right stuff" to succeed. Insurers and patients want practices who have:

- Lower utilization
- Better care coordination
- Better quality
- Better patient experience
- Better patient outcomes
- Lower cost to the insurer and patient

Benchmarking your practice's performance is essential to meeting these expectations and good management will determine whether your practice succeeds or fails.

Digging into Data

The data accumulated during a practice's normal operations are the most valuable, but often underused, management tool. In the course of scheduling, receiving, caring for, and treating patients, along with the subsequent billing processes, a practice generates information that defines its performance. Concurrently, recording revenue and expenses defines its financial status.

Documenting operational and financial performance provides the information needed to identify areas for improvement and by comparing current performance to previous activity lets healthcare leaders anticipate

Chapter 8: The Data Scene

what will happen in the future. Documenting current operations and financial performance is the first step on an organization's road to profitability. Likewise, using practice information to identify areas for improvement and then evaluating its progress initiates the process of continuous improvement which can ensure ongoing success.[1]

With automated data reporting coming from electronic health records (EHR), practice management systems (PMS), payroll systems, accounting reports, telecommunications devices, patient experience surveys and more, practices are awash in data but lacking true business intelligence.[2] Some information, such as financial statements, are required for legal, tax, or financial accounting purposes while other data are collected collaterally with patient services by a scheduling system or EHR. Additionally, the normal course of operations may not have formal recording systems but can generate valuable information that can improve patient service. Utility bills, patient wait times, staffing levels and supply consumption are essential to providing historical information and it is important to establish methodologies to record this information.

Understanding the processes and procedures your organization uses is just as important as the financial and operational data.[3] Unfortunately, identifying how you perform a task is much more complex than recording a financial transaction. Understanding the processes and procedures involved in patient care or business is just as important to improving performance as the quantifiable results reported in financial or performance statistics.

Successful practice managers are proficient in using financial and performance data to make informed decisions and enhance organizational performance. This includes:

- Understanding data sources
- Prioritizing data accuracy
- Setting clear objectives
- Interpreting data
- Knowing relevant metrics
- Possessing financial acumen
- Benchmarking
- Staying compliant

- Communicating effectively
- Embracing continuous learning

By mastering these skills, managers can contribute to the success and sustainability of their medical practices in an increasingly data-driven healthcare environment. According to the *Harvard Business Review*, many healthcare organizations understand that a data-driven approach can help improve patient health incomes, enable faster clinical decisions and improve treatment as well as hospital workflows.[4] Altogether, the comprehensive process of collecting and interpreting information allows you to understand what your organization has done in the past, what it's doing now and what it could be doing in the future.

8.2 Data Sources and Collection

Understanding where data originates, how it is collected and its reliability is the first step in utilizing it effectively. Understanding the accuracy of the data your practice collects is critical to its use. Inaccurate or incomplete data leads to flawed decision-making. Consequently it is critical to continually evaluate data integrity, audit the data collection process and to have an ongoing data quality improvement process to ensure the information used for decision-making is accurate and reliable.

Internal sources of financial and performance data

Ideally, the most accurate and reliable data are from internal sources since you have full control over data collection and the sources of data. Internally, a practice has multiple sources of data that define its financial status and performance.

Financial Statements

The practice's financial statements provide much more information than what is required for legal reporting and tax withholding. Your financial records define the financial condition of your practice at a specific time and provide insight into where practice revenue, expenses and cash flow will be in the future.[5] By reviewing practice financial statements regularly, healthcare leaders can make informed decisions regarding the practice's current financial status, how well their current performance matches the budget forecasted and how well the practice utilized its resources.

Medical groups typically use three basic financial statements to define assets, liabilities and liquidity. For-profit private practices and not-for-profit medical groups use similar financial statements, but the focus and terminology may differ.

- **Income Statement (Profit and Loss Statement):** provides a summary of revenue, expenses and net profit or loss over a specific period, such as a month, quarter or year.
- **Balance Sheet:** presents a snapshot of the practice's financial position at a specific point in time, detailing its assets, liabilities and equity, which demonstrates its overall financial health.
- **Cash Flow Statement:** tracks when cash is generated and when it is paid out during operations, enabling you to manage liquidity and ensuring the practice can meet its financial obligations.

Exhibit 8.1 Sample Balance Sheet

Ray Hospital Balance Sheet September 30, 20X1			
Current assets		**Current liabilities**	
Cash	$8,000,000	Accounts payable	$7,000,000
Net accounts receivable	15,500,000	Accrued expenses	6,000,000
Supplies	3,000,000	Total current liabilities	13,000,000
Total current assets	26,500,000	Long-term debt	45,000,000
Gross plant, property, and equipment	70,000,000	*Total liabilities*	58,000,000
(less accumulated depreciation)	(5,000,000)		
Net plant, property, and equipment	65,000,000	Net assets: Total net assets	33,500,000
Total assets	$91,500,000	*Total liabilities and net assets*	$91,500,000

Practice Management System

The Practice Management System (PMS) records patient information, appointment schedules, billing records and clinical data.[6] The PMS generates the practice's revenue cycle, which provides much more information than just billings and collections. The full revenue cycle provides substantial information describing patient scheduling, revenue streams, reimbursement issues and tracks collection rates providing critical information that can be analyzed to provide information about:

- Patient scheduling and registration describing when a patient schedules an appointment
- The date and time of the patient appointment
- Any copayment paid by the patient
- The procedure codes and diagnostic codes (e.g., CPT and ICD-10 codes) that describe the patient's presenting problem and the procedures performed
- When and how an insurance claim was submitted, the insurer and the gross charges for the services
- Any claim that is denied, the reason for denial as well as when and how the claim is resubmitted
- The claims adjudication explanation of benefits (EOB) generated by the insurer describing the amount covered by insurance and the amount that is the patient's responsibility, including copayments, deductibles and coinsurance
- The amount of contractual adjustments to the gross charge described in the claim adjudication
- The date and amount billed to the patient, including any outstanding balances from previous visits
- The date and amount paid by the patient as well as any discounts or write-offs
- The amount and source of billings declared as bad debt

Electronic Health Record (EHR)

The Electronic Health Records (EHR) system tracks patient demographics, visit volumes, revenue and patient outcomes. According to the Office of the National Coordinator for Health Information Technology,

EHRs are real-time, patient-centered records that make information available instantly and securely to authorized users, and are built to go beyond the standard clinical care collected in a single provider's office.[7] Analyzing EHR data lets you optimize patient care, streamline administrative processes and enhance financial performance.

Regulatory and Compliance Data

Medical practices must comply with numerous government regulations and accreditation standards which were developed to ensure the quality of patient care, protect patient privacy or maintain the integrity of healthcare billing and documentation. Compliance data, including audit reports and adherence to quality measures should be tracked as it also provides valuable insights into practice operations.

Patient Surveys, Social Media Postings and Feedback

Patient surveys and social media postings—along with both unsolicited and solicited patient feedback—provide valuable insights into patient experience and satisfaction.[8] Both objective survey results and unstructured comments let you identify areas for improvement in patient care, communication and service quality. High patient satisfaction is not only essential for patient retention but also for attracting new patients through positive word-of-mouth.

Employee Payroll Systems

A practice receives numerous reports from its employee payroll systems that provide insights into staffing levels, employee costs and attendance. The information, combined with productivity information, provides critical insights into optimizing staffing and can help to identify training needs, recognize high-performing individuals, reduce unnecessary overtime and address performance issues.

There is a wide array of internal sources for financial and performance data that are available to document current and past performance, and provide critical insights into various aspects of practice operations. Regularly analyzing and acting upon this data empowers practice leaders to make informed decisions, improve patient care, optimize financial performance and adapt to changes in the healthcare and business environment.

External Sources of Data

Collecting and evaluating internal data only provides one view of a practice's performance. It is also necessary to understand how the practice compares to its peers. This requires having external sources of unbiased data that can provide perspective. Before we discuss the actual process of comparing internal performance information to external data, it is important to first understand the external sources of data that can be used to compare a practice's performance to peer organizations.

Medical Group Management Association (MGMA)

On a national scale, the Medical Group Management Association (MGMA) has published accurate compensation, productivity and economic performance information since its inception in 1926.[9] MGMA's annual surveys collect information from MGMA members and other medical practices and professionals that are published in the MGMA DataDive Software, an online-based platform with six Data Sets, each focusing on a different aspect of practice performance.[10]

- **DataDive for Provider Compensation:** reports physician and advanced practice provider compensation, retirement benefits, collections, gross charges, total relative value units (RVUs), work RVUs, encounters and other metrics
- **DataDive for Management and Staff:** reports compensation and retirement benefits for practice executives, senior management and employees
- **DataDive for Cost and Revenue:** reports staffing levels, revenue cycle performance, practice revenue, expenses and productivity levels
- **DataDive for Practice Operations:** reports hours of operation, wait times, appointment availability, call volume, employee turnover and other fundamental metrics that show how patients and employees relate to the organization

- **DataDive for Better Performers:** reports the performance of a subset of practices which were selected for having superior results in the DataDive for Cost and Revenue compared to their peers in the areas of operations, profitability, productivity and value
- **DataDive for Procedural Profile:** reports the CPT coding profiles for provider specialties describing how providers code services

Other National Trade and Professional Associations

Practice leaders, physicians and practices may belong to national, regional or local associations such as the American Medical Association, Healthcare Financial Management Association, or physician specialty societies that collect and report quality, performance and compensation data.[11] Those, along with government entities, national accreditation organizations, academic journals, and information gleaned from sources —including patient satisfaction surveys vendors, consulting groups and commercial health insurance companies—can also be helpful in providing best practices on collecting and utilizing existing data streams.

State medical group management associations and state medical societies often conduct employee compensation surveys that focus on the local or regional employment market.[12] Federal and state agencies publish information on multiple areas of interest to practice leaders including national employment levels, wage statistics, Medicare payments, Medicare Physician Fee Schedule (MPFS) data and healthcare quality, including patient safety, clinical performance measures and healthcare utilization metrics. Federal agencies publishing health information include the Bureau of Labor Statistics (BLS), Health Resources and Services Administration (HRSA), Centers for Medicare & Medicaid Services (CMS), Agency for Healthcare Research and Quality (AHRQ) and others.

As part of their mission, national accreditation organizations publish data on healthcare quality, including accreditation and performance measures for healthcare organizations and summaries of accreditation surveys that practice administrators and clinical leaders can use to improve healthcare quality, patient safety, and clinical performance.

These organizations include the Accreditation Association for Ambulatory Health Care (AAAHC), The Joint Commission, the National Committee for Quality Assurance (NCQA) and the Utilization Review Accreditation Commission (URAC).

Commercial health insurance companies often provide reports to medical practices on the utilization of services and reimbursement rates. These reports may include data on the volume of procedures, patient outcomes and revenue performance compared to peers. Academic research and medical journals such as the *New England Journal of Medicine, Mayo Clinic Publications for Medical Professionals and the National Institutes of Health's PubMed Central* also frequently publish data related to clinical outcome, patient satisfaction and best practices in healthcare providing valuable external sources of data for comparisons.[13]

Usually focusing on select practice specialties such as cardiology, consulting groups and for-profit benchmarking companies often collect practice information while providing benchmarking data and analysis tailored to their clients. By comparing one hospital, department, service line, provider group or other aspect with a peer organization, a healthcare provider can determine where it stands and work to undertake improvements.[14]

Most medical practices conduct patient satisfaction surveys, usually contracting with a vendor that specializes in patient surveys. In addition to returning the clients survey results, patient satisfaction survey vendors usually provide comparison reports of the practice's patient satisfaction scores to national or regional averages. As well, the vendors that develop and support EHR or the practice management and billing systems may collect and aggregate information for their clients that provide focused information that has a common collection process.

By collecting financial, performance and quality data internally and evaluating practice information in the context of external sources of data, you gain a better understanding of your practice's financial performance, patient care quality and operational efficiency. Additionally, having external information will help to identify areas for improvement and make informed decisions to enhance your practice's performance.

8.3 Utilizing Data

Before using practice data for management decisions, it is often necessary to manipulate the information so it can be properly interpreted. Most frequently, this involves standardizing or normalizing the data to fit the definitions used by the industry and to accommodate differences in practices.

Standardizing Data to Create Comparison Metrics

Standardizing or normalizing data is the important first step to compare your practice's information to other organizations. According to the Healthcare Information and Management Systems Society, inconsistent and unreliable data can lead to delays in critical patient care and missed opportunities for internal improvement, as well as limitations to monetizing more valuable data.[15] Standardizing creates ratios or percentages to account for changes in your organization over time and also allows you to compare your information to that of other organizations which may be larger or smaller. The most common methods of standardizing practice data involve creating appropriate ratios on either units of input or units of output, or by calculating percentages.

Commonly used ratios calculated "per unit of input":

- Per Full Time Equivalent (FTE) physician
- Per FTE provider
- Per square foot

Commonly used ratios calculated "per unit of output":

- Per patient
- Per Resource-based Relative Value Scale (RBRVS) unit
- Per procedure

Commonly used percentages:

- Cost as a percentage of revenue
- Collections as a percentage of billings
- The percentage of a single payer's patients or payments as a percentage of all payers

The standardizing process involves a simple series of steps.

1. Define the metric and identify its source: Define the metric or performance indicator you want to use. This could be financial metrics (e.g., revenue, profit, expenses), operational metrics (e.g., productivity, customer satisfaction) or other relevant measures. Confirm that the process used to collect data internally is consistent and complies with the definitions established by the organizations publishing external comparison information.

2. Collect the raw data: Identify the internal sources of data and collect the raw metrics that will be used.

3. Select a standardizing factor: Decide on the appropriate unit of input / output or percentage that will create the best ratio that adjusts for the differences in organization size. Identify the internal source of the data that will comprise the denominator of the ratio—i.e., the number of full-time-equivalent (FTE) physicians—and collect the data that will be used to create the denominator for the ratio.

4. Calculate the standardized metric: Divide the raw metric (Step 2) by the chosen normalization factor (Step 3) to calculate the standardized metric. This creates a ratio or percentage that accounts for organization size.

5. Monitor and Update: Standardized metrics should be periodically reviewed and updated to reflect changes in the available external data source or if your practice's size or business strategy changes significantly. This ensures that comparisons remain relevant and accurate over time.

8.4 Key Performance Indicators (KPIs)

Your practice management, accounting and EHR systems generate massive amounts of data that can overwhelm your ability to track and interpret your practice's performance. The problem of data overload is not unique to healthcare, and businesses worldwide have adopted a methodology that identifies the key performance indicators (KPIs) to describe how an organization is performing. By identifying and monitoring the key metrics that are relevant to the success of your practice, you can devote your time to managing performance and not just reading reports.

Since you are managing fewer metrics, identifying the right KPI is critical. KPIs need to reflect the practice's goals and will vary by organization. KPIs need to be observable, achievable, reasonable and aligned with the organization's goals.[16] For example, a not-for-profit community health center may use KPIs that support its patient care mission by measuring total patients and patient experience scores, whereas a physician-owned private practice may want KPIs that measure success as the compensation and benefits of the practice's shareholders. Remember, KPIs will change as the practice and its goals change. Practices evolve over time and may add new services or open additional locations which will necessitate creating new KPIs.

The easiest way to identify the KPIs for your practice is to identify what is key to its success and then identify the metrics available from your EHR, financial, patient accounting or medical information systems. KPIs must be quantifiable (measurable) and the definitions and measurement must be constant over time. KPIs can be either a lagging (e.g., operating cost as a percentage of total medical revenue) or a leading indicator (e.g., new patient registrations) of success.

Prior to using KPIs to measure practice performance it is critical to have executive, physician and staff buy-in so that the KPIs accurately reflect their purpose. Accepting that the KPIs accurately reflect practice success will support using the data for decision making, especially if management uses the KPIs to reduce staffing levels or close programs. Lastly, fewer key metrics are preferred to a multitude of data points so practice leaders can concentrate their attention and observe changes in the KPIs.

Nine KPIs for Financial Success in Medical Groups

Since economic security is fundamental to continued operation, KPIs that measure a practice's profitability and its ability to collect payments and manage expenses are universal.[17] Just nine well-selected KPIs allow you to understand:

- The revenue cycle of recording, billing and collecting for services
- Cost-efficiency
- The bottom line, expressed in the basic formula of total revenue minus operating expense and provider costs

Four KPIs that can assess overall financial performance

Four metrics provide sufficient insight to measure profitability in every practice:

- **Total medical revenue per FTE physician:** Evaluates the total volume of revenue produced by the practice
- **Total operating cost per FTE physician:** Measures the level of operating costs that were consumed in creating revenue
- **Total medical revenue after operating cost and non-physician provider cost per FTE physician:** Reflects the practice's net bottom line before physician compensation
- **Physician compensation:** Is the "bottom line" for independent practices and confirms the ability to match market standards for hospital-owned practices

Four KPIs that can assess the Revenue Cycle

Since a medical practice lives and sometimes dies by its revenue cycle, it is critical to monitor how the inflow of cash from collecting accounts receivable (AR) fuels the practice's financial engine. KPIs based on data from the PMS allow you to assess the most critical functions of the entire revenue cycle: the outstanding amount that needs to be collected, how much of accounts receivable is in danger of being too old to collect, and how fast it is collected and how much of what the practice is owed is collected. You can assess the most critical functions of the entire revenue cycle with four KPIs:

- **Total accounts receivable per FTE physician:** Provides the volume of A/R that needs to be collected
- **AR over 120 days:** Describes how much AR is old and more difficult to collect

Chapter 8: The Data Scene

- **Days of gross charges in AR:** Describes how AR relates to total volume of revenue
- **Adjusted fee-for-service collection percent:** Tells how well the practice collects billed charges

One KPI that can evaluate overall practice efficiency

A single metric can summarize how well a practice converts investments in capital equipment, facilities, human resources, consumable supplies, and technology into revenue.

- **Total operating cost as a percent of total medical revenue:** describes the relationship of total operating costs (all costs not directly related to physician or non-physician compensation or benefits) to revenue. Just as important is its inverse (Total medical revenue as a percent of total operating cost) which describes the operating margin for the practice

Identifying Measures of Healthcare Quality

The authors of MGMA's *DataDive for Cost and Revenue* applied an evidence-based, structured performance measurement methodology to identify measures of healthcare quality for primary care in three principal areas:

1. Access: Ensure the patient has appropriate access to preventive, acute, or chronic healthcare services when needed.

- New primary care patient average wait time in days
- Established primary care patient average wait time in days
- Average 3rd next available appointment in primary care clinics
- Ratio of total inbound patient secure messages to total outbound patient secure messages
- Urgent care utilization rate

2. Patient-healthcare team partnerships: Build a trusting, effective, sustained partnership between the healthcare team, the patient, and his/her caregiver(s) towards shared goals.

- Patient's satisfaction rating of primary care provider
- 2 Day post inpatient discharge contact
- Percent of patients with a documented discussion of stress level

3. Technical quality: Deliver safe and effective care that comprehensively addresses a given patient's psychological, biological and/or psychosocial needs.

- Ambulatory care sensitive conditions (ACSC) hospitalization rate per 1000 patients
- Percent of diabetes patients with poor glycemic control (HbA1c)
- Type 1 Diabetes Composite Score (T1DCS)
- Percent of patients with cardiovascular disease prescribed statin medication
- Percent of patients controlling high blood pressure
- Percent of patients with nephropathy that receive renal testing
- Percent of patients with depression that receive effective continuation phase treatment
- Hospital-wide all cause 30-day readmission rate

8.5 Benchmarking Concepts

Benchmarking involves comparing a medical practice's performance metrics to industry benchmarks or peer practices and helps you understand how your organization measures up against others in terms of financial performance, patient outcomes, or operational efficiency.[18] Benchmarking is an important process that helps identify areas for improvement and can provide valuable insights into best practices.

Benchmarking lets you identify areas where your practice underperforms compared to its peers. This can include financial performance, operational efficiency, quality of care, patient satisfaction or any other relevant metrics. Comparing a practice's performance to its peers identifies areas for improvement and helps set realistic and achievable performance improvement goals.

Chapter 8: The Data Scene

History of Benchmarking

Benchmarking, as a formal business practice, gained prominence in the late 20th century, although its origins can be traced back to medieval times when craftsmen and tradesmen compared their techniques and products to improve quality and efficiency.[19] In the 18th and 19th centuries, the Industrial Revolution saw the emergence of factories and mass production and organizations began to focus on standardizing processes to improve efficiency and quality. According to the Global Benchmarking Network, a formal process for benchmarking performance was created by the Xerox Corporation in the late 1970s, as well as coining the term itself.[20] Xerox used benchmarking to identify best practices in various areas, including manufacturing, sales and customer service which contributed significantly to its success as an international manufacturer. In the 1980s and 1990s, benchmarking gained widespread adoption across manufacturing, healthcare and finance as organizations recognized the benefits of learning from others and implementing best practices to improve their own performance.

Benefits of Benchmarking

Benchmarking standardization also comes with its own list of positives for a healthcare organization. As an incentive for competition, quality improvement, better allocation of resources and improved decision making, benchmarking can be a useful driver.

By adopting best practices and learning from better performing practices, benchmarking helps you stay competitive. You can use it to identify inefficient processes and streamline operations, reduce costs, and enhance productivity. Overall quality can improve when implementing best practices in business, care delivery, quality and patient service. By modeling your practice's processes and procedures on peer organizations recognized for delivering quality services, you will improve care delivery and identify potential risks to patients.

By analyzing benchmarking data, it allows for optimized resource allocation. You can make informed decisions about where to best move those assets, which ensures that staff and other resources are focused on areas that will have the most benefit to your patients and your practice's financial success. Benchmarking also provides valuable data and insights that can guide and improve decision-making. It is the basis for making data-driven decisions, rather than relying on intuition or guesswork.

Types of Benchmarking

Benchmarking is the process of comparing your practice's performance, processes, or practices to a known standard or to other practices to identify areas for improvement. According to BMC Health Services Research, benchmarking has been recognized as a valuable method to help identify strengths and weaknesses at all levels of the healthcare system.[21] It involves the continuous process of measuring and comparing performance internally (over time) and externally (against other organizations and industries). More advanced forms of benchmarking involve determining how the "best in class" achieve their performance levels and using the analysis to change what you do and how you do it (Process Benchmarking).

There are several types of benchmarking and different organizations will tailor their benchmarking process to their needs.[22] Three fundamental types of benchmarking include:

Internal Benchmarking

Internal benchmarking examines a practice's performance over time to identify trends that enable leaders to respond to changes in the environment. Internal benchmarking also involves comparing one part of an organization to another. For example, a practice with multiple branches can compare the performance of one branch with another, or to the average performance of every location. This type of benchmarking can help identify and propagate best practices within an organization while improving consistency across the entire practice.

Competitive Benchmarking

Competitive benchmarking, as the name suggests, involves comparing your performance to peers or to published metrics. The goal is to identify areas where your organization under performs or outperforms similar practices. This type of benchmarking is critical for understanding where to focus management attention and resources.

Strategic Benchmarking

Strategic benchmarking focuses on comparing your organization to entities that are recognized as leaders or "best in class" for their operations. These entities may be in healthcare or from an outside industry but what is important is that the entity is recognized to excel in areas that are relevant to your organization's strategic goals. An example of strategic benchmarking would be to study a nationally recognized hospitality company or hotel chain that excels at providing personalized service and implementing their processes to create a more personalized experience for your patients.

Other Benchmarking Terminology

In addition to the three primary types of benchmarking, other benchmarking terms commonly used include:

- **Performance Benchmarking:** describes comparing overall performance of your practice or its processes against similar organizations or industry standards
- **Process or Functional Benchmarking:** involves comparing specific functions or processes within your organization with "best practices" for performing similar activities
- **Product Benchmarking:** more often occurs in manufacturing and focuses on comparing the quality, features and performance of a product or service with those of competitors or industry leaders
- **Financial Benchmarking:** involves comparing financial performance, ratios and KPIs to national standards, to gain insight into your financial health and efficiency

Describing the Benchmarking Process

Benchmarking performance is a strategic tool that lets you identify areas for improvement, learn from others, set improvement goals and enhance your practice's competitiveness, efficiency, and overall success. It helps you make informed decisions, stay agile in a rapidly changing healthcare environment and demonstrate a commitment to continuous improvement and excellence. According to the American Association for Physician Leadership, effective benchmarking involves a 10-step process that you can use to systematically evaluate your practice's performance against external organizations.[23]

1. Determine what is critical to your organization's success.
2. Identify KPIs that measure your specific objectives for organizational success.
3. Determine sources of internal/external benchmarking data and determine how the data are defined so you can record internal information that is comparable with the benchmark.
4. Measure your performance—gathering internal data from historic records or by collecting concurrent data.
5. Analyze and compare the collected data to identify differences between your organization's performance and the benchmark.

   Compute the difference of your data from the benchmark:
   = Your data − Benchmark
   Compute the percent difference:
   $$= \frac{\text{Your data} - \text{Benchmark}}{\text{Benchmark}}$$

6. Based on the comparison, determine if you need to take action.
7. If you need to take action, identify who does the process best. Identify organizations, both internal (different departments or branches within your practice) or external (other medical practices or industries), to serve as benchmarking models.
8. Determine the best practices and strategies deployed by "better performing" practices that contribute to their superior performance. These can include process improvements, technology adoption, training programs or organizational culture.

9. Implement changes, reassess practice objectives, evaluate benchmark standards and recalibrate measurements.
10. Do it again—benchmarking is an ongoing process, and tracking performance over time allows for continuous improvement. You should continuously monitor and assess performance against benchmarks to understand the impact of the changes and improvements made as a result of benchmarking.

When benchmarking performance, it is important to document the entire process, including the choice of KPIs, findings, actions taken and results achieved. Effective communication of benchmarking outcomes will ensure buy-in from stakeholders and facilitate organizational learning. Before diving into benchmarking, remember:

- Healthcare is a multivariate environment
- Hospital systems are very different than independent practices
- You may need to drill-down to find the best comparison
- Benchmarking provides context for interpreting practice information

Why Your Organization Needs Benchmarking

Benchmarking analyzes your processes in the context of how other organizations and those selected for "better performance" perform the same function. It also lets you understand how your processes are different and what you need to change to improve performance.

Benchmarking helps to identify:

- How others do business
- Whether they are more productive or efficient
- How you can use their methods to improve your performance

Benchmarking can also help:

- Evaluate your strengths and weaknesses
- Analyze your performance over time and compared to peers

- Understand what others are doing so you can learn from the best
- Objectively identify opportunities for improvement
- Convince physicians and staff of the need for change
- Improve decision-making (Evidence-Based Management)
  —Prioritizes improvement priorities

  —Reduces uncertainty and builds confidence

  —Helps explain decisions and supports your management expertise

Benchmarking moves raw data to information and then to actionable analytics

- Practice data alone gives you limited information.
- Practice data in the context of how the metrics change over time or how your practice compares to peers tells you a lot.
- Data starts as raw, unprocessed facts in spreadsheets and databases.
- When data is organized and interpreted, data becomes information.
- The benchmarking process analyzes information and compares practice performance to peers allowing you to make improvements and assess change over time.

8.6 Process Benchmarking

Process benchmarking, also called functional benchmarking, is a systematic and structured approach to analyze and improve how your practice performs key processes and procedures by evaluating what you do compared to how industry leaders perform similar activities. Process benchmarking can be accomplished within an organization or in the context of a formal collaborative of like practices and follows a similar approach as the 10-Step Benchmarking process.

1. Identification of Processes: The first step in process benchmarking is to identify the specific processes or procedures that need improvement.

This could be a part of a larger operation, a departmental process, or a specific task within an organization.

2. Selection of Comparison Information or Benchmark Partners: Once the process to be improved is identified, you need to identify the source of the comparison. The *MGMA DataDive for Practice Operations* contains information on how peer practices are organized to perform certain activities and it breaks out how "Better Performing Practices" are different from other, similar organizations.[24] Another option is to identify a benchmark partner who will share their information. A benchmark partner can be an external organization recognized for their excellence in the specific process or it can be a department or branch internal to your practice that excels in the area being studied. It is also possible that your benchmark partner could be "out of industry."

3. Data Collection: Your organization and its benchmarking partner(s) need to collect relevant data on the process you are benchmarking, which may include process descriptions, time and motion studies, KPIs, quality measurements, costs or other relevant information. Similar data needs to be collected from both the organization and its benchmark partners.

4. Gap Analysis: After data collection, perform detailed analysis to identify gaps or differences between your organization's process and the benchmark partners' processes to recognize how differences in how a process is performed contributes to the difference in outcomes.

5. Understanding Best Practices: Study and analyze the best practices employed by the benchmark partners. This can be accomplished by a site visit to directly observe the processes or by reviewing documentation to understand the methods, tools, technologies and strategies they use to achieve superior results.

6. Determine a Plan of Action: Evaluate what changes need to be made in your processes so you can implement changes.

7. Process Redesign: Devote time to reengineer your existing processes to incorporate the best practices identified from the benchmark partner. This could involve changes in supervisory roles and responsibilities, implementing new technologies, tools, software, changing workflows or in employee training.

8. Implementation: Implement the redesigned process in a segment of your practice or throughout the organization.

9. Monitoring and Measurement: Continue to monitor the newly implemented process using the same metrics and KPIs that were used to identify the areas needing improvement. Regular measurement ensures that the process is performing as expected and achieving the desired improvements. Additionally, study the changes you made internally to ensure that they were fully implemented throughout the practice.

10. Feedback and Continuous Improvement: It is important to obtain ongoing feedback from employees and other stakeholders. Continuous improvement is an ongoing effort to ensure that the process remains efficient and effective over time. Process benchmarking is not a one-time activity, and you should periodically review and repeat the benchmarking process to ensure that your practice remains competitive and aligned with industry best practices. It is also important to document the changes you made and to communicate the effect of the process benchmarking with your physicians and employees so they will remain aware of what was accomplished.

The Benefits of Process Benchmarking:

Process benchmarking is a strategic tool that allows you to identify areas for improvement by comparing your organization's processes to those of industry leaders or internal best practices. It is a structured approach that involves data collection, analysis, redesign, implementation and continuous monitoring that drives organizational excellence and competitiveness. Its benefits include:

- Improved efficiency and productivity
- Enhanced product or service quality
- Cost reduction and resource optimization
- Better customer satisfaction

- Increased competitiveness in the market
- Informed decision-making based on industry best practices
- Opportunities for innovation and continuous improvement

Peer Networks and Management Collaboratives

Process benchmarking can be accomplished independently within your practice, or you can collaborate with other practices to share performance data and best practices. When multiple organizations more formally aggregate their benchmarking activities, they can form a collaborative network or consortium. These peer networks and group collaborations provide their participants valuable insights for performance improvement that may not be available in published reports.

A management collaborative can simply be an informal meeting of similar organizations, or it can be formed through a formal agreement. What is important is that multiple organizations come together to share information, knowledge, resources and expertise to collectively improve processes and procedures. The collaborative approach facilitates exchanging information that fosters innovation, promotes best practices and helps organizations address common challenges. Management collaboratives can be formed to focus only on a specific issue such as may occur when a national organization or government body convenes a study group or they can be long term entities formed by peer organizations that meet periodically.

While informal collaboratives easily form and dissolve as the needs of their members change, formal management collaboratives typically form within a larger health system or by national or regional organizations that create a formal agreement describing the purpose, goals and structure of the collaborative and use the agreement to recruit the organizations that will form the collaborative.

There are a number of common characteristics associated with collaboratives. When a collaborative is created, participating organizations need to identify their common goals, challenges or areas where improvement is needed. The shared interests serve as the foundation for the collaboration and can include areas such as: improving operational efficiency, enhancing customer service, complying with regulatory requirements or addressing industry-specific issues. Collaboratives create a platform for peer-to-peer learning and knowledge sharing so participants can learn from one another's experiences, successes and failures.

A collaborative typically has a governing body or steering committee composed of representatives from member organizations that establishes policies, defines the scope of collaborative activities, and ensures that resources are allocated effectively. Member organizations may have different levels of participation, from active contributors to observers. Similarly, the cost of the collaborative must be shared among its members according to an agreed-up formula. Formal collaboratives typically employ facilitators to oversee the collaborative, organizing meetings, conferences, or online forums for participants to interact and exchange information.

Open and transparent communication and information sharing is essential within a management collaborative as is the free exchange of information and knowledge. Members share data, best practices, case studies, research findings and practical insights. Information sharing can occur through regular meetings, conferences, webinars, online platforms, or working groups.

Management collaboratives frequently involve benchmarking activities where participants compare their organization's performance metrics to those of their peers. They identify areas for improvement and exchange information so the collaborative members can adopt strategies and methods that have proven successful in their peers.

Participants collaborate to solve common challenges and explore innovative solutions, engaging in joint initiatives and projects designed to address shared issues and collectively improve processes and procedures. They also offer opportunities for participants to network and build relationships with others in their field that can lead to future collaborations and partnerships.

Participants provide mutual support and hold one another accountable for achieving specific goals. Periodic evaluations and impact assessments are conducted to measure the effectiveness of collaborative efforts.

This assessment helps determine whether the collaborative is achieving its goals and delivering value to its member organizations.

A management collaborative is a collaborative network where organizations come together to share information and resources to collectively improve processes and procedures. Management collaboratives are flexible structures that adapt to the specific needs and goals of the participating organizations or individuals. They promote a culture of continuous learning, innovation and collective problem-solving while fostering a sense of community and shared responsibility. By pooling knowledge and expertise, management collaboratives address common challenges, drive innovation and achieve better outcomes than its members could achieve on their own.

Benchmarking Quality

While most practice administrators first think of benchmarking in the context of financial, productivity and staffing, benchmarking quality is a critical area for practice success and is essential for delivery of quality patient care.

Additionally, national accreditation organizations such as The Joint Commission and the Accreditation Association for Ambulatory Health Care (AAAHC) require that organizations desiring accreditation must document benchmarking activities that compare key performance measures with similar organizations, with recognized best practices and/or with national targets or goals.[25]

Documentation of a quality benchmarking and continuous quality improvement program is required for accreditation of an ambulatory surgery center. The Federally Qualified Health Center (FQHC) may be mandated for practices that operate as an ambulatory care facility, patient centered medical home, or if the practice is part of a health system.[26]

Benchmarking quality follows a similar process as benchmarking any other facet of a practice.

Determine What to Measure: Assess the importance of clinical outcomes, patient satisfaction and maintaining a safe environment to the practice's success. If the practice is required to maintain formal accreditation as part of its state or federal licensure, then it must comply with the standards for accreditation as failure to maintain accreditation will be catastrophic. Providing quality care in a patient centered environment is critical to long term success but should not result in closure.

Identify Quality Metrics: The most critical aspect of benchmarking quality is to identify what to measure. The metrics can address clinical outcomes, patient satisfaction, safety, efficiency, compliance with accreditation standards, or conforming with federal or state regulations. Ideally the measures should be based on research showing that the measure leads to improved clinical services, that compliance with the measure is associated with desired patient outcomes and that it should have minimal or no unintended adverse consequences.

Define Benchmarks: Determine the benchmarks against which you'll compare your quality metrics. Benchmarks can be set based on national or regional averages, industry standards, or the performance of similar medical practices. In addition to the national accrediting organizations, federal agencies and national organizations such as National Quality Forum (NQF)[27] and the National Committee for Quality Assurance (NCQA)[28] publish quality metrics and establish performance standards.

Measure: Measure your performance and normalize your data to match the benchmark. Collect data related to the identified quality metrics. The source of information may include patient medical records, clinical outcomes, patient surveys, or performance indicators reported in the practice electronic health record. You may need to standardize the data to accommodate the chosen metric. For example, some metrics are normalized by the number of patients to calculate a percent incidence or a per 1000 patient basis. You may also need to adjust the metric for variations in case mix, patient demographics, or other factors that could affect the measure.

Analyze and Compare: Compare your practice data to the benchmark metric to identify differences between your organization's performance and the benchmark and identify where your practice's performance excels and areas where your practice underperformed the standard. The organization that developed the benchmark may also provide national or regional performance standards that you can use for comparison. It is also possible to identify comparison groups, such as peer medical practices, for comparison and to evaluate your practice's performance. In some instances the desired level of performance may be "zero," meaning that any incidence indicates failure, (zero medication error) or as a percentage, (greater than 90% maximum patient satisfaction ratings.)

Determine If You Need to Take Action: For any deficiency from the standard, determine if the difference could result in patient harm (which requires immediate response) or if the issue allows time to research and identify best practices to correct the problem.

Identify Best Practices: If you need to take action, identify who does the process best. The national quality organizations, accreditation organizations, physician specialty boards and other healthcare industry leaders that publish the metrics and benchmarks may also provide information on how to meet or exceed the benchmark. It is also possible that an internal department or branch within your practice may have excellent quality results and can serve as a benchmarking model for other departments.

Implement Changes and Recalibrate Measurements: Quality benchmarks may evolve over time. Periodically reassess your benchmarks to ensure they remain relevant and aligned with the latest industry standards and best practices.

Reset Performance Goals and Identify Improvement Strategies: Establish specific and measurable improvement strategies that may involve changes to clinical protocols, operational processes, staff training or patient engagement initiatives. In areas where significant improvement is needed you may want to create a formal quality Improvement (QI) program: a systematic, formal process including ongoing benchmarking, monitoring, auditing and quality improvement studies.

Monitor Progress and Do It Again: Implement changes, evaluate benchmark standards, recalibrate measurements and track progress toward meeting quality performance goals. Quality benchmarking needs to be ongoing and tracking performance over time is a key component of continuous quality improvement.

As your quality benchmarking program continues, it is important to periodically share your benchmarked quality results and improvement progress with your staff, patients and other stakeholders. Transparency in reporting fosters trust and accountability and allows you to engage your staff to celebrate success while gaining insights from patients on their perceptions of the practice.

8.7 Practice in Action

You are the administrator of a 20-doctor independent multispecialty practice and are concerned that the practice's financial performance is lagging. As you prepare for an upcoming meeting with the medical group president and executive committee, you want to understand specifically where the practice is succeeding and where it needs improvement. You pull the latest financial and revenue cycle information from your practice's financial records and billing system and identify the Key Performance Indicators that will allow you to analyze practice revenue, expenses, staffing, revenue cycle and productivity. You also extract information from the MGMA *DataDive for Cost and Revenue* so you can benchmark your performance.

Use KPIs to assess the practice's performance and identify areas that require your management attention by answering the following questions:

1. What is happening in the practice revenue, expenses and profits?
2. What is happening in the practice revenue cycle?
3. How productive are the practice's physicians?
4. Is the practice properly staffed?
5. How does your practice compare to other physician-owned multi-specialty groups?
6. How bad a problem is this?

7. As the practice administrator, where do you want to focus your attention?
8. Do you need to immediately revise your resume and look for another position—or is the problem solvable?
9. What are your courses of action?

Even a cursory investigation of the key data points listed here will help give an objective overview of the directions your practice needs to pursue in order to get the financial performance back on target. KPIs are instrumental in validating and guiding a path to recovery.

8.8 Summary

Modern medical practices generate millions of pieces of data about patient visits, tests and every stage of the revenue cycle. Learning to interpret and use that data to improve internal processes and optimize expenditures can help ensure future success.

To summarize, here are some key takeaways:

- Identify both internal and external sources of financial and performance data, and the best ways to collect those sources.
- Raw data can then be standardized to create comparison metrics, from FTEs to RBRVSs.
- Key performance indicators (KPIs) can help assess overall financial performance, track the revenue cycle and evaluate overall practice efficiency.
- Benchmarking against industry standards or other practices can demonstrate how your practice compares to others.
- Internal, competitive and strategic benchmarking use different models to measure success, while process or functional benchmarking takes a more systematic look at the internal mechanisms in your practice.

In the next chapter, we will discuss the importance of marketing in healthcare while providing helpful marketing strategies for your medical practice.

Notes

1. ASQ. https://asq.org/quality-resources/continuous-improvement
2. AMA. https://www.ama-assn.org/practice-management/claims-processing/how-select-practice-management-system
3. RLDatix. https://resources.rldatix.com/en-us-blog/top-5-types-of-healthcare-policies-and-procedures
4. HBR. https://hbr.org/sponsored/2023/08/innovation-in-data-driven-health-care
5. Withum. https://www.withum.com/resources/medical-practice-accounting-101-understanding-your-financial-statements/
6. Definitive Healthcare. https://www.definitivehc.com/resources/glossary/practice-management-system
7. HealthIT.gov. https://www.healthit.gov/faq/what-electronic-health-record-ehr
8. NIH. https://www.ncbi.nlm.nih.gov/pmc/articles/PMC8156131/
9. MGMA. https://www.mgma.com/overview-mission
10. MGMA. https://www.mgma.com/datadive
11. HFMA. https://www.hfma.org/
12. Massachusetts Medical Society. https://www.massmed.org/About/State-Medical-Societies-in-the-U-S-/
13. NIH. https://www.ncbi.nlm.nih.gov/pmc/
14. Syntellis. https://www.syntellis.com/the-definitive-guide-to-healthcare-benchmarking
15. HIMSS. https://www.himss.org/resources/revolutionizing-healthcare-through-data-standardization
16. MGMA. https://www.mgma.com/articles/data-mine-measuring-success-finding-the-right-metrics-to-optimize-the-revenue-cycle
17. MGMA. https://www.mgma.com/articles/flooded-by-data-while-thirsting-for-information
18. Gregory S. Feltenberger and David N. Gans. "Benchmarking Success: The Essential Guide for Medical Practice Managers, 2nd Edition.," Medical Group Management Association, 2017
19. The Benchmarking Group. https://benchmarking.com.au/insights-trends/the-history-of-benchmarking/
20. Global Benchmarking Network. https://www.globalbenchmarking.org/index.php/whats-benchmarking/development-of-benchmarking/
21. BMC Health Services Research. https://bmchealthservres.biomedcentral.com/articles/10.1186/s12913-022-07467-8
22. NIH. https://pubmed.ncbi.nlm.nih.gov/10139084/

Chapter 8: The Data Scene

23. AAPL. https://www.physicianleaders.org/articles/benchmarking-healthcare-steps-improvement
24. MGMA. https://www.mgma.com/datadive/practice-operations
25. AAAHC. https://www.aaahc.org/uploads/2023/01/AAAHC-v42-Handbook-MDS_FINAL.pdf
26. HealthCare.gov. https://www.healthcare.gov/glossary/federally-qualified-health-center-fqhc
27. NQF. https://www.qualityforum.org/Home.aspx
28. NCQA. https://www.ncqa.org/

Chapter 9

Marketing Strategies for Medical Practices

By: Jennifer Thompson, MHA

9.1 Introduction

Effective marketing is no longer a luxury—it's a necessity for medical practices to thrive and better serve their communities. The rise of consumerism, changing patient expectations, and the advancement of digital health have heightened the importance of a strong digital front-door strategy to attract and retain patients. Practice managers and doctors face a myriad of challenges—hospital acquisitions, the influence of private equity and declining reimbursement rates—all of which contribute to an increasingly complex and competitive environment. To navigate these obstacles successfully, you need a strategic approach to marketing that not only attracts new patients but also fosters long-lasting relationships and adapts to the evolving needs of the healthcare market.

This chapter is designed to provide you knowledge and tools to effectively market your practice in this dynamic landscape. By exploring the key components of a successful digital front-door strategy, you'll learn how to position your practice for growth, build a strong online presence and create a patient experience that sets you apart from the competition. Whether you're a seasoned practice manager or a doctor looking to enhance your marketing efforts, this chapter will equip you with the insights and strategies you need to succeed. Let's dive in and discover how you can make a lasting impact on your patients and your community.

9.2 The Importance of Healthcare Marketing Strategy

Beyond traditional advertising, referral outreach and community involvement, healthcare marketing involves building connections, fostering trust and delivering information to patients in need. A well-executed marketing strategy will help you:

- **Increase Patient Awareness:** Effective marketing ensures that your practice's name is recognized within your community, enabling patients to find and choose your services when in need easily.
- **Build Trust, Better Reviews and Credibility:** Through educational content and patient testimonials, you can establish your practice as a reliable source of healthcare information and demonstrate your commitment to patient well-being.
- **Enhance Patient Engagement:** By connecting with patients through digital platforms, you can provide support, share health tips and encourage healthier lifestyles.
- **Boost Patient Retention and Referrals:** A comprehensive marketing strategy can foster stronger patient relationships, increase patient loyalty and generate more referrals through positive word-of-mouth.
- **Adapt to Industry Trends:** With the evolution of technology and patient expectations, an up-to-date marketing approach ensures your practice remains relevant and competitive in the ever-changing healthcare landscape.

In the face of increasing competition and a rapidly changing healthcare landscape, understanding the importance of healthcare marketing is essential for medical practices looking to attract and retain patients, foster long-lasting relationships and ultimately thrive in today's market.

Healthcare consumers increasingly rely on online platforms for health-related information and decision-making, with 58.5% of U.S. adults using the Internet to look for health or medical information.[1] Your online presence is how you will reach and engage with potential patients.

Sixty percent of patients consult search engines first when finding a new doctor or researching a referred physician.[2] You must invest in search engine optimization (SEO) and targeted digital marketing efforts to ensure you are easily discoverable by potential patients. This includes optimizing your presence on digital directories such as Google Business pages, which can significantly improve visibility and make it easier for patients to find essential information like contact details, hours of operation and patient reviews.

> **60% of patients consult search engines first when finding a new doctor or researching a referred physician (Hohensee & Zeitzer, 2021).**

Email marketing remains a powerful tool for healthcare communication, boasting an average open rate of 21.48% and a click-through rate of 2.69%.[3] This allows you to nurture relationships with existing patients, keep them engaged and promote relevant services.

Social media has also become a significant source of health information, with over 80% of internet users aged 18-49 reporting that they seek health information on social media platforms.[4] You should leverage this trend by maintaining a social media presence, sharing content and building trust with your target audience.

Adopting a digital front-door approach to marketing, which focuses on creating a seamless and engaging online experience for healthcare consumers, is necessary in today's competitive and consumer-driven market. By improving and focusing on the customer experience, including marketing efforts, you can potentially achieve a revenue increase of 20% over five years, with a 30% decrease in cost to serve.[5]

Artificial intelligence (AI) is beginning to disrupt various industries, and healthcare will be no exception. AI-powered tools and technologies are being used to streamline processes, improve patient outcomes and enhance the overall healthcare experience. As AI advances, medical practices that embrace these technologies and integrate them into their marketing strategies will be better positioned to meet healthcare consumers' evolving needs and expectations.

A comprehensive healthcare marketing strategy that leverages digital platforms, search engines, digital directories, email marketing, social media, and AI-driven technologies is essential for your practice to attract, engage, and retain patients. Embracing a digital front-door approach and prioritizing the customer experience can help you position your practice for long-term success.

Unique Challenges and Considerations in Healthcare Marketing

Your role in healthcare marketing extends beyond promoting your services; you must navigate the delicate balance between ethics, patient privacy and trust in an increasingly digital world.

Trust forms the bedrock of your relationship with patients, and with 65% of healthcare seekers turning to Google before their doctor, establishing a trustworthy online presence has become both a growing challenge and a necessity.[6] As healthcare consumers increasingly rely on online platforms for health-related information and decision-making, your digital presence needs to instill confidence and credibility.

The rise of social media and online reviews has created a continuous feedback loop on the performance of your physicians and your practice. Patients now have the power to share their experiences, both positive and negative, with a broad audience. This transparency has made trust more essential than ever before but also made it easier to lose. A single negative review or a mishandled social media interaction can quickly erode the trust you have worked to build.

The services you promote can directly impact an individual's health and well-being. Your marketing must be accurate, transparent, and guided by integrity while reaching new and returning patients. This requires a balance between leveraging the power of digital platforms and maintaining the trust and privacy of your patients.

Ultimately, trust is the key to success in healthcare marketing. It improves outcomes for everyone involved—patients, providers and the healthcare system. As you navigate the digital landscape, keeping trust at the forefront of your strategies is paramount. This means monitoring and managing your online reputation, addressing patient concerns and delivering quality care that aligns with your marketing messages.

9.3 Understanding Your Target Audience

Speaking directly to your audience can help you differentiate your practice, showcase your expertise and demonstrate your commitment to meeting their specific needs. Personalized messaging drives increased engagement, laying the foundation for lasting relationships with your patients and the long-term growth of your practice. To speak directly to your audience, start with thorough research. Leveraging data from website analytics, social media insights and patient surveys can help you understand your audience's preferences, behaviors and pain points. Then craft personalized narratives that address their concerns and demonstrate your ability to meet their needs. It's not about reaching the most people; it's about reaching the right people with the right message.

Conducting Effective Market Research

Many providers rely heavily on patient data. Age, location, income—these broad demographic strokes can be misleading. The 35-year-old professional mother's priorities may differ from those of the 37-year-old single woman, despite similar data profiles. You can't just collect data. You need to seek insights. Build your strategy by looking at patient profiles and identifying different audiences within these demographics that could be attracted to your practice. Ways to conduct market research include:

- **Surveys and Questionnaires**: These can be used to collect demographic information, preferences, and healthcare needs directly from current and potential patients. They can

be deployed online or in person, offering quantifiable data to shape your marketing strategies.
- **Focus Groups:** By organizing sessions with a small, diverse group from your target audience, you can observe their attitudes, perceptions and expectations regarding your practice. This qualitative research provides insights that surveys alone may not uncover.
- **Digital Analytics:** Tools like Google Analytics or social media insights offer a window into the online behavior of potential patients. By analyzing patterns in website traffic, social media engagement and search queries, you can understand what prospective patients seek online.
- **Patient Interviews:** One-on-one conversations with current or potential patients can provide deep, personal insights. These interviews can uncover motivations, challenges and desires that inform your marketing approach.
- **Competitor Analysis:** Studying your competitors' strategies, strengths and weaknesses can reveal opportunities for differentiation. Look at their marketing messages, services offered and patient feedback to identify areas where you can stand out.

Market research is an ongoing process of listening, learning and adapting. As your audience evolves, so should your understanding of them. You can develop a comprehensive picture of your target audience by combining quantitative and qualitative insights. This understanding should guide your marketing efforts, ensuring your messages resonate and your services meet real needs. Market research is about building empathy by seeing the world through the patients' eyes.

Establishing patient personas of your target audience is a good tool for framing your marketing plan. Use the data of already existing clients to create a potential client—including age, sex, occupation, activity level, lifestyle, etc. This profile then becomes a real individual, someone who is not currently a patient but who fits the bill of your current patient demographic. This becomes the profile of who your marketing is targeting. Practices that integrate patient personas into their marketing efforts experience a 30% ROI on their marketing expenditure.[7]

Chapter 9: Marketing Strategies for Medical Practices

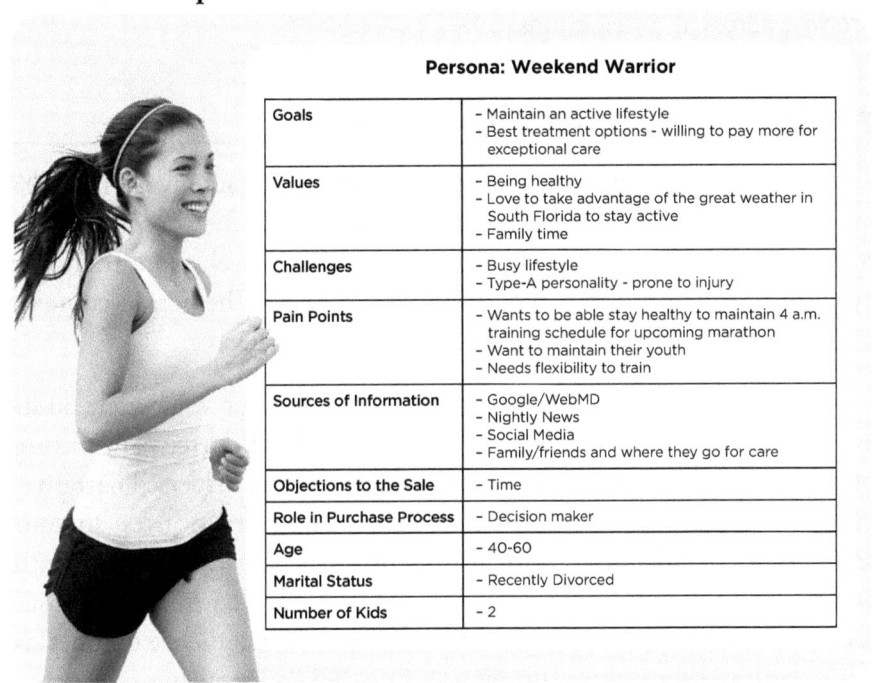

Exhibit 9.1 Sample Patient Persona

Persona: Weekend Warrior	
Goals	- Maintain an active lifestyle - Best treatment options - willing to pay more for exceptional care
Values	- Being healthy - Love to take advantage of the great weather in South Florida to stay active - Family time
Challenges	- Busy lifestyle - Type-A personality - prone to injury
Pain Points	- Wants to be able stay healthy to maintain 4 a.m. training schedule for upcoming marathon - Want to maintain their youth - Needs flexibility to train
Sources of Information	- Google/WebMD - Nightly News - Social Media - Family/friends and where they go for care
Objections to the Sale	- Time
Role in Purchase Process	- Decision maker
Age	- 40-60
Marital Status	- Recently Divorced
Number of Kids	- 2

Analyzing Market Trends and Competition

Many providers view competition through a commoditized lens. They study rivals' offerings and pricing, then position themselves as a slightly cheaper, convenient alternative. But true differentiation arises from identifying and meeting unmet needs. By prioritizing communication, empathy and personalized care, your practice can focus on delivering an exemplary patient experience at every touchpoint.

Advertising advancements in treatments and technology is important, but it's most effective when coupled with a clear articulation of how these innovations will meet the specific needs of your audience in ways other practices cannot. Your unique offerings become narratives, transforming your services from interchangeable options into something distinct. Engage with your patients to find these opportunities for differentiation. Identify the gaps in the current landscape and position yourself to fill them. Build a brand that stands for something meaningful in the minds of your patients, then consistently communicate and deliver on this brand promise across all interactions.

9.4 Developing a Strong Brand Identity

Your brand extends far beyond face-to-face interactions. With 50% of patients placing as much trust in online reviews as they do in personal recommendations, it is clear that modern patients seek more than just proximity or pedigree when choosing a provider.[8] They crave context, nuance and a brand that speaks to and works for them.

Your brand is not solely what you promote but what your audience perceives. It's the imprint left in the minds of current and future patients—a collection of every interaction, review and dispersed narrative. How you make someone feel shapes their willingness to invest in your services over a competitor's. Patients seek providers they can trust and with whom can build long-lasting relationships. To succeed in this environment, practices must pursue a connection with their audience that builds trust and fosters meaningful relationships beyond securing temporary transactions. Building a solid healthcare brand in the digital age requires a multi-faceted approach that includes:

- Consistently delivering high-quality care that aligns with your brand promise.
- Actively managing your online reputation by monitoring and responding to patient reviews and feedback.
- Creating valuable, personalized content that addresses your target audience's needs and concerns.
- Leveraging social media and other digital platforms to engage with your audience and build trust.
- Ensuring that every touchpoint—from your website to your waiting room—reflects your brand values and creates a positive patient experience.

By prioritizing brand-building and patient connection in the digital age, providers can differentiate themselves in a crowded market, attract new patients and foster long-lasting relationships that improve health outcomes.

Crafting a Compelling Brand

Your brand is a promise and expectation you set for every interaction with a patient. The brand is baked into everything you do. When you keep that promise, people become loyal patients that praise and refer your practice to others, and they'll stick around because you've delivered a cohesive experience that resonates. Key components of a strong brand identity include:

- **Mission and Values:** Clearly articulate what your practice stands for and the core values that guide your patient care. This helps patients understand what makes your practice unique and why they should choose you.
- **Visual Identity:** Your logo, color scheme, and typography should reflect your practice's personality and values, making a memorable impression on current and potential patients. Consistency in visual elements across platforms enhances brand recognition.

Developing a Unique Value Proposition

Your value proposition answers the question every patient asks: "What's in it for me?" It's not merely a list of services or credentials—it cuts through and connects with the real human need.

Whether it's understanding and empathy during a difficult time, expertise to overcome a chronic issue or preventative care to stay healthy, you need to be clear about improving the patient's situation. A focused value proposition makes brand ambassadors out of satisfied patients. Components of a successful value proposition include:

- **Uniqueness:** Identify what sets your practice apart. This could be your cutting-edge treatment options, exceptional patient care or specialized expertise.
- **Clarity:** Communicate your value proposition in simple, understandable terms. Avoid medical jargon to ensure your message is accessible.
- **Relevance:** Tailor your value proposition to meet the needs and concerns of your target audience. It should address the key benefits your patients can expect to receive.

Designing a Professional and Visually Appealing Brand Identity

Your brand isn't just a look—it's a signal. In healthcare, those signals go beyond aesthetics. The visuals say who you are and what you believe. They're how people decide if you're the right fit for their needs. Does your website radiate expertise and empathy, or is it cold and detached? Impressions are often made before the first appointment is booked. In a world of ever-expanding choices, people spend less time evaluating and more time filtering.

According to Amra & Elma, 82.8% of US-based patients used search engines to find a healthcare provider.[9] An informative and visually inviting website serves as the digital front door to your practice, encouraging potential patients to explore your services and engage with your practice. Ensure your brand identity resonates with your target audience with:

- **Professional Design:** Invest in high-quality designs for your logo, website and marketing materials. A professional appearance reinforces the quality and reliability of your healthcare services.
- **Consistency:** Ensure your visual branding is consistent across all platforms and materials. Consistency helps build recognition and reinforces your brand identity in the minds of your audience.
- **Engagement:** Use visual branding to tell a story about your practice. Incorporate images and testimonials that reflect your patients' positive experiences to create an emotional connection with your audience.

Exhibit 9.2 Visual Brand Identity—Logo Concept

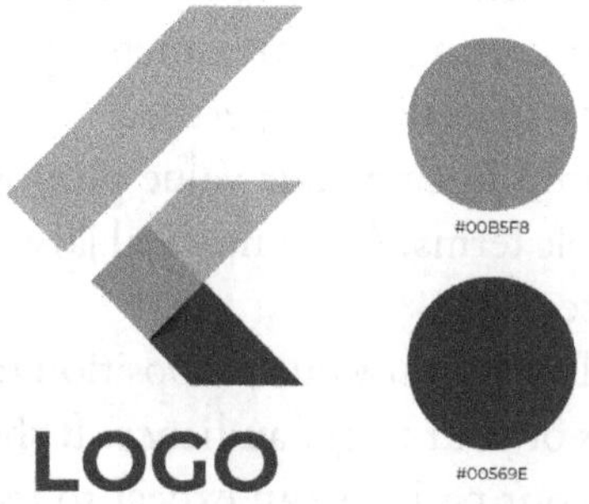

9.5 Online Presence and Your Website

Having a digital presence means being where your patients are and making it easier for them to find and connect with your practice. This digital shift doesn't diminish the value of traditional methods but complements them, opening new avenues for patient engagement and practice growth. Below are some quick tips to enhance your online presence.

- **Optimize Your Website:** Your website is often the first point of contact with potential patients. Ensuring it's mobile-friendly is a top priority, as over 59% of web traffic now comes from mobile devices.[10] A fast-loading site can significantly reduce bounce rates, with a one-second delay in load time increasing the bounce probability by 32%.[11]
- **Verify Your Practice Information:** Consistent and accurate information across platforms enhances your credibility and helps with search engine rankings. Incorrect information can lead to a loss of patient trust and missed appointments.
- **Maximize Google My Business (GMB):** An optimized GMB profile can increase your practice's visibility in local searches. Patients will find your practice through your GMB, as 84% of customer searches for businesses are discovery searches, while only 16% are direct searches.[12]
- **Active Social Media Engagement:** Social media isn't just for sharing content; it's for building relationships. With over 4 billion people using social media worldwide, platforms like Facebook and X offer a vast audience for your practice to engage with.[13]
- **Highlight Reviews on Doctor Rating Sites:** Positive reviews on doctor rating sites can influence potential patients' decisions. 72% of patients say they preferred choosing providers rated four out of five stars or higher.[14]
- **Get Help from Healthcare Marketing Experts:** Engaging with healthcare marketing experts can further streamline this process, allowing you to focus on providing top-notch care while growing your practice online.

Building an Effective Website

Your digital strategy should prioritize your website's design and usability. A well-crafted website should showcase your services and expertise while delivering an easy-to-use and informative experience. Key elements of an effective website include:

- **Patient Experience (PX):** Ensure your website is easy to navigate and book appointments with a structure that guides visitors to the information they seek without frustration.
- **Responsive Design:** Your site must perform flawlessly across devices, especially mobile phones, where many users now access the internet.
- **Speed:** Website loading times should be under three seconds; slow-loading pages deter potential patients and negatively impact your search engine rankings.
- **Educational Content:** Provide valuable, accessible information about your services, conditions treated and patient care. Highlighting patient testimonials and case studies can also build trust with prospective patients.
- **Local Search Engine Optimization:** Provide content information and highlight your location on service pages.
- **Resources and Videos:** Dedicate part of your website to celebrating your providers, staff, and great patient experiences with video testimonials to build trust with potential patients checking out your practice online.

Exhibit 9.3 Sample Website User Behavior Metrics

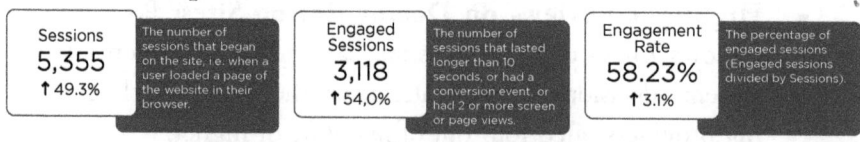

Sessions		Engaged Sessions		Engagement Rate	
5,355 ↑49.3%	The number of sessions that began on the site, i.e. when a user loaded a page of the website in their browser.	3,118 ↑54.0%	The number of sessions that lasted longer than 10 seconds, or had a conversion event, or had 2 or more screen or page views.	58.23% ↑3.1%	The percentage of engaged sessions (Engaged sessions divided by Sessions).

According to WebFX, 90% of online users will switch to a competitor's website following a poor user experience.[15] A high-quality, user-friendly website keeps your new patient and retention rates up.

How to Do Content Marketing

The internet has flipped the script on how people discover and engage with your practice. A blog that demystifies chronic conditions, videos addressing common fears and concerns, and guides that empower people in their health journeys—all of these are tools at your disposal. By providing real insights that move people along their path, you earn an engaged audience that chooses to avail themselves of your expertise because you've helped them so much already. Effective content marketing can:

- **Establish Expertise:** Share your knowledge through blog posts, infographics, videos, and articles on topics relevant to your audience. This demonstrates your expertise and helps in answering common patient questions and concerns.
- **SEO Benefits:** Regularly updated content improves your website's visibility on search engines, making it easier for potential patients to find you.
- **Social Engagement:** You can engage your audience through educational and informative content, encouraging them to interact with your practice through comments, shares, and other social media actions.

> **82.8% of US-based patients used search engines to find a healthcare provider (Amra & Elma, 2023).**

Utilizing Social Media Platforms

Social media platforms can bolster your online presence, allow you to interact with your audience and amplify your content—this increases your visibility and accessibility. Use these platforms to share updates, post educational content and engage with your community. Through regular posts and interactions, you can build a community around your practice, fostering a sense of loyalty and trust among your followers. Social media offers direct lines of communication with your audience, allowing for feedback and insights into their preferences and concerns.

Online Advertising Strategies

Online advertising, including pay-per-click (PPC) campaigns and social media ads, can boost your practice's visibility and attract new patients. Digital ads can be highly targeted based on demographics, interests, location, and user behavior, ensuring your message reaches the relevant audience. The effectiveness of online advertising campaigns can be precisely measured, allowing for optimization and adjustment to improve ROI. Digital advertising campaigns can be adjusted or halted based on performance, market conditions, or budget considerations.

Exhibit 9.4 A/B Testing Case Study

Test A — Get Ahead of Allergies, Book Your Test Today / Schedule Allergy Test Online

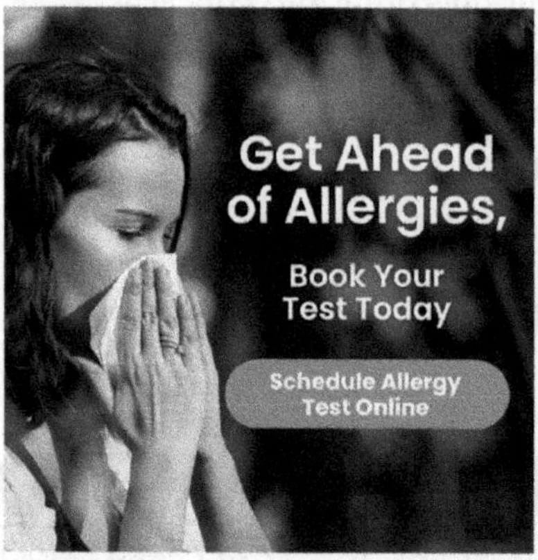

Test B — Top-Rated Allergists. Say goodbye to allergy & sinus problems *for good*. It's only one quick allergy test away. Book Now

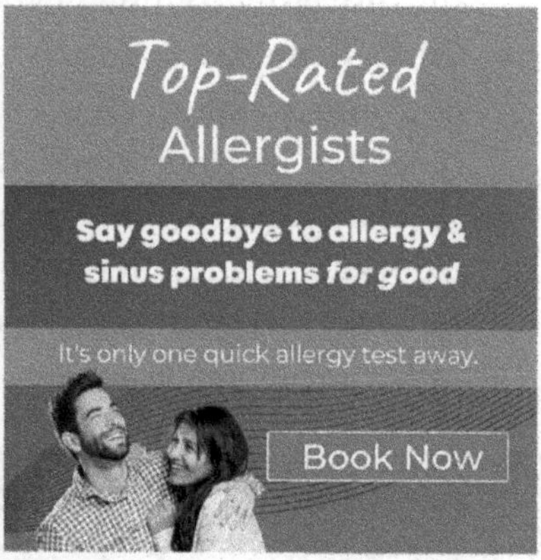

CASE STUDY

An ENT practice used an allergy-focused Google Ads campaign to attract patient prospects seeking local allergists. Assets included Google Ads (text), display ads (visual), social ads (visual) and YouTube pre-roll ads (video). Various visual styles and ad copy were tested to find the message that resonated most with the audience. Some platforms, like Facebook and Google, allow you to A/B test within the platform and then the platform intuitively delivers the ad that performs best.

RESULTS

- 2,395 conversions into patients
- 13.8% conversion rate
- 536,093 impressions
- $39,837 spend

Local Search Engine Optimization

Search Engine Optimization (SEO) can heighten your website's visibility on search engines like Google. It entails fine-tuning your site's content and structure to secure higher rankings in search results for keywords. Local SEO is promising, as it amplifies your impact within your patients' communities. Identify and incorporate keywords that potential patients might use to find services like yours. Optimize your website for local search queries to attract patients in your geographical area. This includes listing your practice on Google My Business and other local directories. Earning backlinks from reputable sites within the healthcare industry can enhance your site's authority and search ranking.

How Long Until You See Growth?

You've been taught that marketing is a magic bullet. Invest heavily and voila—new patients start pouring in. But what if that's backwards? The practices that get marketing right don't see it as a short-term campaign. It starts by giving the patients you already have a seamless experience—one they'll remark about online. Then, you build a digital home that's true to your values. You engage in the places where your audiences are listening and learning. Genuine growth can happen in 30 days. But remember, by becoming a practice people admire and relate to, you'll be too established to outgrow.

9.6 Patient Referral Programs and Relationship Management

While marketing campaigns and promotions can be effective, the most potent growth engines are often overlooked. According to Referme IQ, 65% of new business originates from referrals, making it clear that word-of-mouth recommendations are required for the success of any provider.[16]

Providers must focus on delivering exceptional patient experiences at every touchpoint to harness the power of referrals. This means providing high-quality personalized care, creating a welcoming environment, using clear and empathetic communication with patients, following up after appointments, and encouraging satisfied patients to share their experiences with others.

By prioritizing patient satisfaction, providers can tap into the power of referrals and create a self-sustaining growth engine for their practice. In a world where patients have more choices, earning their trust and loyalty is the key to long-term success.

Building Relationships with Referring Physicians and Healthcare Professionals

The success of a thriving referral program lies in the relationships between your practice and fellow healthcare professionals. These connections are built on trust, open communication and mutual advantage. Strategies for developing these relationships include:

- **Regular Communication:** Keep referring physicians informed about their patient's progress and treatments. This demonstrates your commitment to collaborative care.
- **Networking and Professional Engagement:** Participate in local and professional healthcare associations. This engagement allows for face-to-face interactions with potential referrers.
- **Providing Value:** Offer educational resources or seminars that benefit referring physicians and their practice. This positions you as an expert and enhances your relationship.

Enhancing Patient Experience and Satisfaction

A positive patient experience cultivates word-of-mouth referrals. Satisfied patients are inclined to advocate for your services among their friends and family, creating organic growth for your practice. According to Etactics, there's a 4% improvement in patient lifetime value for every 1% increase in retention.[17] Enhancing the patient experience involves several key areas:

- **Personalized Care:** Tailor the patient experience by recognizing their needs and preferences. Personalization can range from greeting patients by name to customizing their treatment plans.

- **Efficient Service:** Minimize wait times and simplify administrative processes to respect patients' time. Efficiency in these areas contributes to overall satisfaction.
- **Quality Interactions:** Ensure every interaction with your staff is friendly, informative, and supportive. The quality of these interactions weighs heavily on a patient's overall perception of their care.

Implementing a Patient Referral Program

A structured referral program incentivizes patients to refer others to your practice. These programs may incorporate referral incentives but always adhere to ethical guidelines and compliance standards regarding incentivizing referrals. Implementing an effective referral program includes:

- **Clear Communication:** Inform patients about your referral program through your website, social media or during appointments.
- **Ease of Referral:** Make the referral process easy. Provide referral cards or a simple online form.
- **Acknowledgment and Appreciation:** Follow ethical guidelines to show appreciation for referrals, whether through a thank you note, a small gift or public recognition.

9.7 Community Engagement and Local Marketing

Your participation in the community and local marketing are indispensable components of a holistic marketing strategy. Your practice can be a local pillar of value by taking community engagement as serious work—it's showing up consistently to listen, teach and be visibly human where stakeholders live. Your engagement with the community is about cultivating connections. Hosting or participating in health fairs, community events, and local sponsorships offers avenues to interact with potential patients and other local businesses.

Community events and health fairs can showcase your services, treatments, and expertise directly to potential patients in a non-clinical setting, making your practice more approachable. By participating in and sponsoring community activities, you demonstrate a commitment to the local community, fostering trust and goodwill. These events provide opportunities to network with other local businesses and organizations, opening doors to potential partnerships and referrals.

Strategies for Effective Community Engagement

Choose events that align with your practice's specialties and target audience. For example, a pediatric practice might participate in local school health fairs, while an orthopedic clinic could benefit from sponsoring a community 5k run. Provide information or services at events, such as free health screenings, educational seminars, or interactive workshops. This approach attracts attendees and positions your practice as a valuable resource within the community. Utilize your website, social media channels and local media to promote your involvement in community events. Effective promotion ensures maximum visibility and attendance.

Local marketing tactics can increase your practice's visibility and draw new patients. Strategies may include local SEO or pay-per-click (PPC) advertising campaigns to secure placement in local search and map results. Advertising in local publications, listing your practice in local directories, and actively participating in local online forums and social media groups can enhance your local presence.

Ensure your practice's website is optimized for local search queries related to your specialties. Include your location in key SEO elements like titles, meta descriptions and content. Add locations, directions and local content to your website to enhance your local SEO. Advertise in local newspapers, radio or community bulletins. Tailor your messaging to highlight the unique aspects of your practice and its commitment to the community.

While growth doesn't occur overnight, local event marketing can attract new patients quickly. However, developing and executing these campaigns takes time. Active community engagement and strategic local marketing should enhance a medical practice's reputation and establish a robust patient base. Establish a timeline to achieve your objectives and manage expectations accordingly.

9.8 Patient Testimonials and Online Reviews

Patient testimonials and reviews shape how you are seen. Firsthand stories of care and outcomes often matter more than marketing slogans. Testimonials are unpaid endorsements motivated by goodwill—they're reminders of the humans impacted by your work. Prospective patients should see them not as PR fluff but as windows into the experience they'd like to have. While testimonials provide valuable perspectives, it's important to balance these with objective criteria such as a provider's credentials and experience.

How to Address Negative Feedback

Negative reviews are inevitable, but managing them correctly mitigates their impact and demonstrates a commitment to quality and satisfaction. Here's how to approach negative feedback:

- **Respond with Empathy:** Acknowledge the review, apologize for any negative experience and avoid defensive responses.
- **Move the Discussion Offline:** Offer contact information for a private conversation, ensuring the reviewer feels heard without airing grievances publicly.
- **Take Action and Follow Up:** Assess the feedback for validity, make necessary improvements and consider contacting the reviewer after the resolution.

Negative ratings can stem from not soliciting positive patient testimonials and reviews. Certain reviews may be spam or unrelated to your practice. It's important to proactively monitor your reputation while also showcasing positive content and encouraging the sharing of patients' positive experiences. Enhancing and protecting your practice's reputation involves several steps:

1. **Encourage Positive Sharing:** Facilitate the process for patients to leave positive reviews by providing direct links to review sites and requesting feedback post-visit.
2. **Monitor Your Online Presence:** Set up alerts for mentions of your practice to respond promptly to new reviews,

maintaining an active engagement with patient feedback. Monitor popular healthcare reputation sites like Doctor.com and Healthgrades.com.

3. **Accuracy and Engagement:** Update your practice's information online to avoid credibility loss due to inaccuracies. Engage with your community through events and social media to bolster your practice's visibility and connection to patients.

4. **Create Positive Content:** Regularly publishing positive patient testimonial videos, news about your practice, and blog content can push your practice up in search results and provide social media content. This can reduce negative content and increase trust in your practice, even if you have a recent negative rating.

Thoughtfully engaging with patient reviews and encouraging patients to share their positive experiences online can enable your practice to build a reputation that attracts and retains patients. Here are strategies to facilitate this:

- **Ask at the Right Time:** The best time to ask for a review is when a patient expresses satisfaction with their care. A simple, "We're glad to hear you had a positive experience. Would you mind sharing this feedback online?" can be effective.
- **Make it Easy:** Provide clear instructions or links to where patients can leave reviews, such as on your website, Google My Business, or healthcare review sites. The easier it is, the more likely they will follow through.
- **Highlight the Importance:** Explain to patients how their testimonials can help others make informed healthcare decisions. Understanding the impact of their reviews can motivate patients to share their experiences.

Authentic patient stories resonate strongly with potential patients. Showcasing patient testimonials with permission can be a powerful tool in attracting new patients. Dedicate a section of your website to patient testimonials while also incorporating them into brochures, emails and social media posts.

9.9 Measuring and Analyzing Marketing Performance

Grasping the impact of your marketing efforts is essential for steering your growth in the right direction. As you craft your marketing strategy, it's vital to set clear goals, identify KPIs, and harness marketing data to fine-tune patient acquisition and engagement. There's a direct link between meticulous performance analysis and the successful attraction of new patients. Measure and analyze your performance to ensure effectiveness and maximize your return on investment (ROI). This clarifies what's working and highlights areas that need tweaks or enhancements.

Setting Marketing Goals

Your first step in measuring marketing performance is to set clear, achievable goals. These goals should be specific, measurable, attainable, relevant, and time-bound (SMART). For example, you might aim to increase patient appointments by 10% in six months or boost your social media following by 20% within a year. By setting precise targets, you can gauge the success of your efforts and make the necessary adjustments.

Identifying the Marketing KPIs of Your Practice

KPIs exist to guide your assessment of the efficacy of your strategies. Picking the appropriate KPIs offers insights into your marketing performance and aligns your expectations and trajectory. Common KPIs in healthcare marketing include:

- **Website Traffic:** The number of visitors to your practice's website, which can indicate the effectiveness of your online presence and SEO efforts.
- **Patient Booking Rate:** How many patients book appointments online, and how often? You can also see how many patients book online compared to patients attending a consultation or booking a procedure.

- **Patient Acquisition Cost:** The total cost associated with acquiring a new patient. It helps assess the efficiency of your marketing spending.
- **Conversion Rate:** The percentage of website visitors or social media followers who take a desired action, such as booking an appointment.
- **Patient Satisfaction Scores:** Patient feedback provides insights into the quality of the service and areas for improvement.
- **Referral Rates:** The number of new patients referred to your practice, indicating the success of referral programs and patient satisfaction.

Analyzing Marketing Performance

With clear goals and KPIs, your next step is consistent review and analysis of these metrics. Leveraging tools such as Google Analytics to scrutinize website performance, social media analytics to gauge engagement and reach, and patient management systems to monitor appointments and referrals, you'll find invaluable data for refining your strategies. Regular analysis allows you to:

- **Identify Trends:** Understanding long-term patterns can inform strategic decisions.
- **Optimize Strategies:** By knowing what works well and what doesn't, you can allocate resources more effectively and adjust tactics.
- **Demonstrate ROI:** Clear metrics demonstrate the value of marketing investments to stakeholders.

Measuring and analyzing your marketing performance guides your decision-making process. This may entail reallocating focus to channels yielding greater effectiveness, fine-tuning messaging to resonate more with your target audience, or utilizing new technologies and tactics to stay ahead of the curve.

Tracking performance is necessary when refining strategies. Implementing analytics tools, establishing conversion tracking, and generating reports require significant time investment. However, this investment can help you navigate marketing strategy with clarity and make informed decisions that lead to more effective patient acquisition and engagement.

9.10 What's Next & Future Trends in Healthcare Marketing

As we look towards the future of healthcare marketing, it's impossible to predict exactly what lies ahead. The rapid pace of technological advancements and the constantly shifting market dynamics make it challenging to say with certainty what the landscape will look like in the coming years. However, change is inevitable and it's up to you to be prepared for whatever the future may hold.

While we can't know for sure what the future has in store, we can make educated guesses based on the trends we're seeing today. Emerging technologies like artificial intelligence, machine learning and blockchain are already beginning to revolutionize personalized patient care, data security, and marketing efficiencies. As these technologies continue to evolve and become more widely adopted, they have the potential to completely transform the way you connect with your patients and deliver care.

Another trend that is likely to shape the future is the increasing empowerment of patients. As patients become more informed and engaged in their own care, they will increasingly dictate the future of healthcare delivery. They may demand greater convenience, transparency, and personalization in their care experiences, and it will be up to you to find ways to meet or exceed their expectations.

While the uncertainty of the future may feel daunting at times, it's important to remember that change also brings opportunity. By staying attuned to the latest trends and technologies, and by remaining flexible and adaptable in your approach to marketing, you'll be well-positioned to navigate whatever challenges and opportunities the future may bring.

Advanced Strategy for Medical Practice Leaders

Adapting to Technological Innovations

At the forefront of healthcare marketing's evolution is technological utilization. Among the most promising frontiers is AI integration. According to Statista, the anticipated investment in AI within the healthcare sector will soar to $188 billion in the US by 2030.[18] AI could reshape how healthcare practices tailor and customize their marketing initiatives, ultimately enhancing patient experiences and outcomes. Key areas where AI and other technologies are set to make an impact include:

- **Personalized Patient Journeys:** Leveraging data analytics and AI to tailor marketing messages and interactions based on individual preferences and behaviors.
- **Automated Patient Engagement:** Using chatbots and automated messaging to provide information, reminders, and support to patients, enhancing their experience.
- **Predictive Analytics:** Applying AI to predict patient needs and behaviors, allowing practices to offer services and information, improving patient health outcomes.

Want to test AI for your medical practice? Below are examples of AI prompts to help you further explore some of these marketing ideas for your practice:

- How to Perform a Medical Website SEO Audit
- Outline Search Ad Campaign to Target Treatments and Conditions for My Practice
- Write a Step-by-Step Guide to Build an Email List for My Practice
- Outline Design and Copy to Send a Monthly Newsletter to My Patients
- How Can My Practice Utilize Geofencing Ads to Convert New Patients
- Write a Script and Storyboard a Video to Feature a Physician at My Practice
- Outline a Backlink Building Strategy to Grow Organic Search Traffic for (Procedure or Service)

- What Should I Add to My Practice's Profile for Google Business Profile Optimization
- Outline Content for OTT & C-TV for My Practice
- What Lead Magnets Would Be Best to Bring in Patients for (Procedure/Service/Doctor)
- Outline a LinkedIn Strategy to Connect with Local Physicians for Referral Growth

Embracing Digital Transformation

The trajectory of healthcare marketing's future hinges on embracing digital avenues, from telehealth platforms to social media engagement, guaranteeing accessibility and convenience for patients. This transformation demands a strategy that reaches patients on their chosen platforms, anticipates their needs and incorporates new methods for delivering healthcare.

Authentic human connections grow more pronounced in this age where we are born with a computer in our palm. The landscape of the future necessitates an approach combining technological progress with genuine empathy and understanding. Elements such as storytelling, patient testimonials and community involvement retain their role in fostering meaningful relationships with patients.

The incorporation of predictive analytics into marketing strategies marks a new frontier. By examining data patterns and patient behaviors, you can anticipate needs, tailor communications, and elevate patient experiences. The future promises a targeted approach, where efforts are calibrated to align with individual patient journeys. This methodology brings about deeper engagement and fosters a sense of personalized care that resonates with patients.

Sustainability and Social Responsibility

The future of marketing strategies will extend beyond patient care to address broader sustainability and social responsibility concerns. Patients increasingly favor providers who commit to environmental stewardship and community well-being.

It's important to recognize that the future of marketing strategies will extend beyond patient care to address broader sustainability and social responsibility concerns. Today's emerging patients favor providers who commit to environmental stewardship and community well-being. By weaving these values into your marketing strategy, you align with patient sensibilities and contribute to a healthier, more conscientious society. This approach emphasizes incorporating ethical considerations and social impact into your brand narrative. In doing so, you demonstrate your commitment to fostering a better community and environment.

9.11 Practice in Action

Bruce, the new marketing coordinator for Peak Orthopedics, is driven to make a significant impact by creating meaningful connections with patients, understanding that successful marketing goes beyond merely promoting services.

Identifying Core Identity and Patient Personas

Bruce's first task is to identify the strengths and core identity of Peak Orthopedics. He notes the practice's innovative treatment approaches, convenient urgent care services and cutting-edge facilities. However, he realizes that many competitors tout similar features and he needs to dig deeper to differentiate Peak Orthopedics. He aims to uncover what truly sets the practice apart and what values underpin their patient care philosophy.

To create a targeted marketing plan, Bruce begins by establishing patient personas. He analyzes data from existing patients, focusing on demographics such as age, sex, occupation, activity level and lifestyle. This analysis reveals common trends among middle-aged athletes, young professionals and elderly patients. Bruce creates detailed profiles for each group to tailor marketing efforts to their specific needs. These personas help in crafting relevant and compelling campaigns that attract new patients and build strong, lasting relationships, ensuring Peak Orthopedics remains a preferred choice in the community.

Chapter 9: Marketing Strategies for Medical Practices

Differentiation Amidst Competition

When a nearby hospital launches a new orthopedic line, Bruce focuses on differentiating Peak Orthopedics through personalized, family-like care and specialized expertise. He enhances the patient experience by simplifying appointments and follow-up care, offering a seamless experience compared to larger hospital systems. Bruce promotes Peak Orthopedics' advanced technology and successful patient outcomes through targeted, cost-effective campaigns and a robust digital presence. Strengthening community ties through outreach programs and expanding the referral network ensures a steady flow of new patients. Bruce remains agile, monitoring the competitive landscape and patient feedback to adapt his strategies and maintain Peak Orthopedics' distinct position.

Crafting a New Brand Identity

Bruce sets out to craft a new brand identity based on his gathered knowledge from patient feedback, competition analysis, and industry trends. He crystallizes the unique value proposition as "Peak Orthopedics: Providing Treatment and Care That Feels Like Family." Collaborating with a graphic designer, Bruce works on visual elements and creates a brand voice that is empathetic and supportive. He establishes a brand guide defining logos, colors, fonts and tone to ensure consistency. A soft rollout allows for immediate feedback, enabling adjustments before a full launch. Throughout the process, Bruce ensures that the brand stays true to its value proposition.

Enhancing Online Presence

With the brand identity solidified, Bruce focuses on amplifying it online. Partnering with a web design firm, he transforms Peak Orthopedics' website into a modern, user-friendly hub that provides a warm, family-like experience. Bruce optimizes SEO and enhances Peak's Google Business Profile to increase online visibility. He employs distinct strategies for each social media platform, developing a content calendar to maintain engagement and consistency. Targeted paid social campaigns showcase compelling patient stories and the unique value proposition, quickly extending Peak Orthopedics' family-like reputation online. This cohesive multi-channel approach strengthens Peak Orthopedics' identity and expands its reach both online and offline.

Building a Robust Referral Network

Bruce then turns his attention to building a robust referral network. He targets local providers like physical therapists and primary care physicians, setting up a patient referral program with online forms and thank you cards. Through informal gatherings and appreciation events, he strengthens personal relationships with referrers. This helps ensure Peak Orthopedics stands out by providing a best-in-class referral experience and fostering meaningful connections, becoming the preferred choice despite the new hospital competition.

Amplifying Local SEO and Patient Testimonials

Bruce optimizes Peak Orthopedics' directory listings and Google Business Profile to amplify local SEO, pushing the practice to the top of hyper-local search results. Geo-targeted social media ads and patient testimonials within their service radius help make Peak's name instantly recognizable in the community. Bruce solidifies Peak Orthopedics as a friendly, familiar orthopedic family woven into the fabric of the community through hyperlocal initiatives.

He also focuses on amplifying patient testimonials and online reviews. By making it easy for patients to leave positive reviews through post-visit prompts and submission links, and showcasing "Patient Spotlights" through professional videos and photos, Bruce ensures a constant stream of authentic patient voices validating Peak Orthopedics' family-like, attentive reputation. This multi-pronged approach leads to an influx of five-star reviews and glowing testimonials, boosting key metrics like website traffic and new patient rates.

Sustaining Growth through Measurable Goals

Bruce is committed to sustaining the progress made. He sets clear, measurable goals to ensure ongoing growth, identifying critical KPIs such as patient acquisition rates, social media engagement metrics, and web traffic conversions. Regular monitoring and monthly review meetings with his team allow for analyzing progress and making necessary adjustments. By sharing detailed data and insights with leadership, Bruce ensures alignment with the organization's goals, fostering a collaborative environment that drives continued success and growth for Peak Orthopedics.

9.12 Summary

The future of healthcare marketing is dynamic and full of opportunities. By staying adaptable and embracing emerging technologies, you can elevate patient engagement and optimize operational processes. The focus should remain on delivering personalized, empathetic care while leveraging digital tools to enhance accessibility and convenience. Prioritizing compliance, sustainability, and social responsibility will build trust and foster long-lasting patient relationships. Navigating the complexities of consumerism, changing referral patterns, and the competitive nature of hospital acquisitions and payer involvement requires a strategic approach. Smaller practices must focus on their unique strengths, maintain a solid online presence, and continuously adapt to industry trends to thrive in this challenging environment. By doing so, they can secure their place in the healthcare market and continue providing exceptional patient care.

To summarize, here are some key takeaways:

- A well-executed marketing strategy will help your practice increase patient awareness, engagement and retention while building trust and credibility.
- Understand your target audience by conducting effective market research. In addition to patient surveys and focus groups, establishing patient personas can help frame your marketing plan with data that defines your target audience.
- Building a solid healthcare brand in the digital age requires a multi-faceted approach from medical practices to not only stand out in a crowded market, but to also attract new patients and foster long-lasting relationships that improve health outcomes.

- By prioritizing patient satisfaction, providers can tap into the power of referrals and create a self-sustaining growth engine for their practice. The success of a thriving referral program lies in the relationships between your practice and fellow healthcare professionals.

In the next chapter, we will discuss the role that health information technology plays in effective healthcare operations. We will cover health IT's importance in operational efficiency, improving patient outcomes and supporting informed decision-making.

Notes

1. CDC. https://www.cdc.gov/nchs/products/databriefs/db482.htm
2. P3 Practice Marketing. https://www.p3practicemarketing.com/insights/the-top-6-ways-patients-search-for-doctors-online
3. Digitals Medical. https://digitalismedical.com/blog/healthcare-marketing-statistics/
4. Market.us Media. https://media.market.us/social-media-in-healthcare-statistics/
5. McKinsey & Company. https://www.mckinsey.com/industries/healthcare/our-insights/marketing-in-healthcare-improving-the-consumer-experience
6. CharityRx. https://www.charityrx.com/blog/the-shifting-role-of-influence-and-authority-in-the-rx-drug-health-supplement-market/
7. Adfire Health. https://adfirehealth.com/blog/how-to-create-detailed-hcp-personas-free-hcp-personas-template/
8. BrightLocal. https://www.brightlocal.com/research/local-consumer-review-survey/
9. Amra & Elma. https://www.amraandelma.com/healthcare-marketing-statistics/
10. Exploding Topics. https://explodingtopics.com/blog/mobile-internet-traffic
11. Instant Page Builder. https://instant.so/blog/how-does-website-speed-impact-conversion-rates
12. Gitnux. https://gitnux.org/google-my-business-statistics/
13. Statista. https://www.statista.com/statistics/278414/number-of-worldwide-social-network-users/
14. PatientEngagementHIT. https://patientengagementhit.com/news/72-of-patients-view-online-reviews-when-selecting-a-new-provider
15. WebFX. https://www.webfx.com/blog/marketing/marketing-stats/
16. Referme IQ. https://www.refermeiq.com/referral-marketing-statistics/
17. Etactics. https://etactics.com/blog/patient-retention-statistics
18. Statista. https://www.statista.com/topics/10011/ai-in-healthcare/#topicOverview

Chapter 10

Advanced Health IT Strategies for Medical Practices

By: Katie Nunn, MBA, CMPE

10.1 Introduction

The integration of Health Information Technology (health IT) has increasingly become a necessity for modern medical practices. From streamlining administrative tasks to improving patient care outcomes, the importance of health IT cannot be overstated. This chapter explores advanced strategies tailored for medical practices to harness the full potential of health IT, navigating through its benefits and challenges to optimize healthcare delivery.

Health IT stands as the cornerstone of modern medical practices, revolutionizing the way healthcare is delivered, managed and experienced. Its importance lies not only in enhancing operational efficiency but also in improving patient outcomes and satisfaction. With electronic health records (EHRs), telemedicine and health analytics becoming integral components of healthcare delivery, medical practices are increasingly reliant on health IT to meet the demands of a rapidly evolving industry.

However, the adoption and implementation of health IT comes with its fair share of challenges. From initial and ongoing costs and interoperability issues to concerns regarding data security and privacy, medical practices encounter various obstacles along the path to integration. Understanding these challenges is crucial for developing effective strategies that mitigate risks and maximize benefits.

An MGMA Stat poll from March of 2023 said that 74% of groups reported an increase in IT expenses in the past year.[1] With security breaches on the rise and increased dependence on IT, we will continue to see increases in this area. However, we are also seeing gains in efficiency that are helping to offset these expenses.

This chapter provides an overview of the benefits and challenges associated with health IT implementation in medical practices. By examining the transformative potential of health IT, we aim to highlight its role in enhancing patient care, optimizing workflows and facilitating informed decision-making. Moreover, we will confront the barriers that impede successful implementation, offering insights into overcoming these obstacles through strategic planning and resource allocation.

By exploring the importance of health IT in modern medical practices, examining its benefits and challenges, and outlining key objectives, this chapter serves as a comprehensive guide for practitioners and healthcare administrators seeking to advance their Health IT strategies. Through informed decision-making and strategic implementation, medical practices can harness the full potential of health IT to deliver high-quality, efficient, patient-centered care in an increasingly digital era.

10.2 Electronic Health Records

Twenty-five years ago, the most commonly asked question in any medical practice was "Where's the chart?" The amount of time that healthcare workers spent trying to answer that question was as surprising as the number of places one would look to find the chart. One problem that EHRs have solved is we no longer have to search offices, cars, breakrooms, dictation stacks, homes, etc. to find the chart. The use of EHRs, once considered a tough transition for practices, is now being implemented by healthcare providers as early as training. The generation of providers that had to make the change from paper to EHR may still have apprehension about its current wide use. Understanding this apprehension is key in understanding how to make it better. According to David N. Gans, MSHA, FACMPE: "Many EHRs were sold on the concept of being a paperless solution; however, first-generation EHRs essentially automated a paper medical record. The reality today is not much different, in that EHRs have become increasingly complex and have undone the promise of administrative simplification."[2] Here we will look at some of those reasons and address ways that you can counter that in your own practice.

User Interface and Usability

Many EHR systems have complex user interfaces that are not intuitive or user-friendly. Users often have to navigate through multiple screens and menus to find the information they need, which can be time-consuming and frustrating. Additionally, EMR systems may not be customized to suit the workflow of individual medical practices, leading to inefficiencies and resistance from doctors who prefer more streamlined processes.

While getting EHR vendors to make changes to their system is possible, it is often not a very quick solution to this problem. We would always recommend submitting an enhancement request for anything that you feel would make your EHR better. If the EHR vendors don't know, they will certainly never make that change and the more complaints they have the more likely they are to address that issue. However, the more practical solution to this problem is training. Many users of EHR systems get very little training when they first start using the system and then often never get follow-up training. This makes it a challenge to use it to its full potential. In an MGMA stat poll from November 2023 we learned that 35% of practices listed EHR usability as a top tech priority.[3]

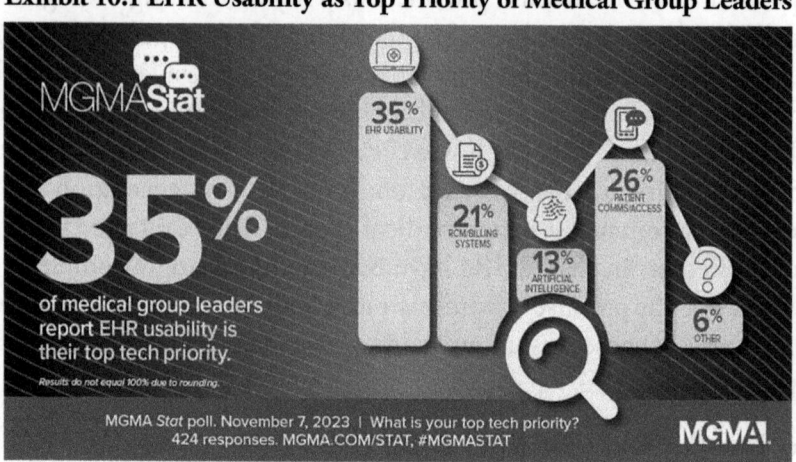

Exhibit 10.1 EHR Usability as Top Priority of Medical Group Leaders

MGMA Stat

35% of medical group leaders report EHR usability is their top tech priority.

Results do not equal 100% due to rounding.

- 35% EHR USABILITY
- 26% PATIENT COMMS/ACCESS
- 21% RCM/BILLING SYSTEMS
- 13% ARTIFICIAL INTELLIGENCE
- 6% OTHER

MGMA Stat poll. November 7, 2023 | What is your top tech priority? 424 responses. MGMA.COM/STAT, #MGMASTAT

MGMA

Time Consuming Data Entry

EHR systems often require extensive data entry, including documenting patient encounters, entering orders for tests and medications, and updating patient records. Providers may feel burdened by the amount of time spent on administrative tasks, which can detract from their ability to focus on patient care. Moreover, the need to input large amounts of data can contribute to provider burnout and dissatisfaction with the system.

As previously mentioned, training providers in all the tools that the EHR has to offer is key. Many systems come with the ability to make short lists, templates, and other shortcuts to help make documentation easier, but many providers don't know these tips and tricks, so they struggle daily with documentation burden. It can be hard to schedule formal trainings for busy providers, but you can pass out a tip or a trick at each provider meeting that you have or send out a monthly email with some tips and tricks so that your team is always learning something new. Also, encourage your providers to share their useful tips with each other. Ask the efficient documenters in your office for guidance on how they stay so efficient and share that with the other members of your team.

AI is also becoming a more prevalent tool in the EHR world. Some systems are starting to have ambient listening devices that record data into the chart while the provider is talking to the patient. The system is smart

Chapter 10: Advanced Health IT Strategies for Medical Practices

enough to recognize the patient's voice versus the provider's voice and it adds documentation to the chart appropriately. This can be a huge time saver and would be less expensive than a scribe. If the EHR system that you have doesn't come with an AI feature, there are also third-party companies that will interface with EHRs so you can still have that functionality.

Interoperability Issues

Despite efforts to standardize EHR, interoperability remains a significant challenge in healthcare. EMR systems may not always communicate effectively with other systems used by hospitals, clinics and other healthcare providers. This can lead to difficulties in accessing patient information from different sources, potentially compromising patient safety and continuity of care. Providers may become frustrated when they encounter barriers to accessing critical patient data in a timely manner.

In an MGMA article titled "It's Time to Plan the Funeral for Fax in Healthcare," Skyler Kent said, "A significant amount of effort and resources has been put into digitizing medical records, and the lack of interoperability is creating more mundane tasks. Anytime a record must be faxed, the receiver must transcribe the information into their EHR, which takes time and is human error prone. Last year when I moved across the country, I changed health providers for the first time in my life. My medical record was more than 300 pages long, resulting in me filling out my medical history two times by hand and verbally to my provider in addition to the 300-plus pages I gave them. All this despite my entire record since birth already being digitized by my previous provider."[4]

Kent goes on to add, "If I get a new phone, I can connect it with my old phone and all my contacts will be moved from one to the other; why can't my medical history be done in a similar fashion? Then there is the financial imperative to achieve such ease of use: communication deficiencies can cost a 500-bed hospital more than $4 million a year."

To navigate these hurdles, physician practices can employ several strategies:

- **Middleware Solutions:** Middleware is software that acts as a bridge between an operating system/database and

225

applications. Investing in middleware solutions can bridge the gap between disparate systems, enabling data translation and interoperability.
- **Standardized Data Exchange:** Advocating for standardized data exchange formats and protocols within the healthcare community can foster interoperability improvements at a systemic level.
- **APIs:** Application programming interfaces (APIs) are software intermediaries that allow two applications to communicate with each other. Utilizing APIs can facilitate data sharing between EHR platforms, allowing for smoother integration and interoperability.
- **Increased Use of Open Source:** In an MGMA article titled "Navigating the Constantly Evolving Cybersecurity Threat Landscape," John Squeo and Vikram Sukthankar write, "The benefits of open source, including fast implementations and low cost, are extensive and why it can be found across the healthcare IT ecosystem today."[5]
- **Partnering with Vendors and Stakeholders:** Fostering collaboration and partnerships with EHR vendors and health IT stakeholders can encourage the development of interoperable solutions tailored to the specific needs of physician practices.

By implementing these strategies, physician practices can mitigate interoperability challenges and enhance the efficiency and effectiveness of patient care delivery.

10.3 Health Information Exchange

Health Information Exchange (HIE) is a crucial component of modern healthcare systems, facilitating the electronic sharing of patient health information among healthcare providers and organizations. At its core, HIE aims to enhance care coordination, improve patient outcomes, and streamline healthcare delivery by ensuring timely access to comprehensive and accurate patient data across disparate systems. This section explores the concept of HIE in depth, examining its benefits, challenges, as well as legal and privacy considerations.

Chapter 10: Advanced Health IT Strategies for Medical Practices

What is HIE?

HIE refers to the electronic movement of health-related information among various healthcare stakeholders, including hospitals, clinics, physician practices, laboratories, pharmacies and public health agencies. HIE enables the secure sharing of patient data, such as medical history, laboratory results, medication records, diagnostic images and treatment plans, in a standardized format regardless of the originating source or platform. While HIE has many benefits, there may not be an HIE in your area, or not all local medical facilities may be sharing data on the HIE level. As far as data sharing is concerned, the healthcare industry is comparable to cell phone networks, but imagine if you could only call or text with people that were on your same carrier.

Benefits of HIE

HIE enables healthcare providers to access a comprehensive view of patients' health information across different care settings, facilitating better care coordination and informed decision-making. This is particularly beneficial in cases where patients receive treatment from multiple providers or transition between healthcare facilities. Access to up-to-date patient information through HIE helps healthcare providers avoid medication errors, adverse drug interactions, and unnecessary procedures, ultimately improving patient safety and health outcomes. HIE can also reduce redundant tests, paperwork, and administrative burden by streamlining data exchange and eliminating the need for manual data entry. This leads to greater operational efficiency and cost savings for healthcare organizations.

HIE supports public health initiatives by enabling timely reporting of communicable diseases, outbreaks and other health trends to public health agencies. This facilitates early detection, response and containment of public health threats. Some practices are required to have interfaces with local or state health departments for vaccines and for case reporting for certain illnesses to be compliant with merit-based incentive payment systems (MIPS). HIE also empowers patients to actively participate in their healthcare by granting them access to their electronic health information, fostering transparency, shared decision-making and patient-centered care. As mentioned, this is also a MIPS requirement for many practices to have a patient portal that gives patients access to their health information. Some portals work with more than one EHR system allowing the patient to have information from multiple practices in one place; however, many do not which means that the patient may have to have multiple portals if they see multiple doctors.

Challenges of Health Information Exchange

Despite efforts to standardize data formats and protocols, interoperability remains a significant challenge in HIE, as healthcare systems often use disparate technologies and data standards. This can impede seamless data exchange and interoperability among different EHR systems and healthcare organizations. Another issue is that many health systems still feel that healthcare data is proprietary and are only willing to share what is mandated by government agencies like CMS. HIE involves the sharing of sensitive patient health information, raising concerns about data privacy, confidentiality and security. Unauthorized access, data breaches, and identity theft are potential risks associated with HIE, necessitating robust security measures, encryption, authentication and access controls to safeguard patient data.

HIE operates within a complex legal and regulatory landscape governed by laws such as the Health Insurance Portability and Accountability Act (HIPAA) in the United States. Compliance with privacy, security, and consent requirements, as well as navigating state-specific regulations, can pose challenges for HIE initiatives. Establishing and maintaining HIE infrastructure, governance, and operations require significant financial investments. This is the foremost reason that we don't have more HIEs that are functioning in the United States.

Legal and Privacy Issues in Health Information Exchange

HIE entities must comply with the HIPAA regulations, which govern the privacy, security and confidentiality of protected health information (PHI). HIPAA establishes standards for data encryption, access controls, auditing, breach notification and patient consent requirements. "Commonly referred to as release of information, the failure to handle it appropriately could be quite costly. Even if the medical practice executive does not serve dually in this role, ultimately the protection of a patient's PHI is the responsibility of the medical group, and by default the medical practice executive. Understanding the Standards for Privacy of Individually Identifiable Health

Information (Privacy Rule) of HIPAA, as well as the 21st Century Cures Act is crucial to know which information can and cannot be released with a release of information request, as well as the time constraints for releases. The penalties for not complying with the myriad standards and requirements can be financially detrimental to your medical practice."[6]

Patient Consent and Authorization

Patient consent and authorization play a crucial role in HIE, as individuals have the right to control the sharing of their health information. HIE initiatives must adhere to HIPAA regulations regarding patient consent for disclosing PHI, including opt-in or opt-out mechanisms and patient preferences for data sharing.

Data Security and Encryption

Protecting health information from unauthorized access, disclosure, or misuse is paramount in HIE. HIE entities are required to implement robust security measures, such as encryption, access controls, authentication, and audit trails, to safeguard PHI during transit and storage.

HIE holds great promise for transforming healthcare delivery by facilitating seamless data exchange, care coordination and patient engagement. However, realizing the full potential of HIE requires addressing key challenges related to interoperability, privacy, security, legal compliance and financial sustainability. By implementing robust governance frameworks, security measures, and patient consent mechanisms, HIE initiatives can navigate these complexities while maximizing the benefits of electronic health information exchange for improved patient care outcomes.

10.4 Telemedicine, RPM and RTM

In recent years, the healthcare industry has experienced a significant transformation due to advancements in technology, particularly in the realm of telemedicine and remote patient monitoring (RPM). Remote therapeutic monitoring (RTM) is the newest of the three to enter the healthcare scene but promises to have a huge impact. These innovations are reshaping the way healthcare is delivered, offering new opportunities for improving patient outcomes, enhancing access to care and optimizing healthcare management. This comprehensive exploration dives into the growing importance of telemedicine and RPM, strategies for integrating telemedicine into medical practices, leveraging RPM technologies for better patient outcomes, and overcoming barriers to adoption while maximizing the benefits of these technologies.

The Growing Importance of Telemedicine and RPM

Telemedicine has become a crucial component of modern healthcare delivery. The COVID-19 pandemic has accelerated its adoption, highlighting its potential to maintain continuity of care while reducing the risk of infection transmission. Telemedicine offers numerous benefits, including increased access to healthcare services, convenience for patients, and cost savings for both patients and providers. Telemedicine has limitations since you can't touch or examine a patient physically; however, some types of visits are perfect for telemedicine as an option. With talk therapy or medication checks, mental health visits are often perfect for telemedicine. The patient can take less time away from work or school and receive care in private.

Exhibit 10.2 Common Uses for Telehealth[7]

FOLLOW-UP CARE	BEHAVIORAL HEALTH	OVERCOMING TRANSPORTATION BARRIERS
• Patients on treatment protocols who need close follow-up care and multiple visits to ensure compliance and manage medication • Care for chronic and complex conditions, including virtual consults on lab results, symptom triage, lifestyle management, and remote patient monitoring (RPM) check-ins • Post-operative wound care • Group education consults with prediabetic and diabetic patients on healthy eating, exercise, and wellness tips	• Address shortages in local or on-site mental health services in rural or underserved populations by connecting patients to a specialist. • For routine follow-ups with anxiety, depression, and ADHD patients who are adjusting to new medications • Routine virtual psychotherapy appointments	• Access care from the convenience of the patient's home • For patients who face mobility barriers and lack a caregiver or assistance with transportation to the doctor's office • Urgent care for established patients with low-risk, infectious diseases, such as conjunctivitis or urinary tract infection • For long-term patients who are temporarily relocated out of state • Pre-orthopedic surgery preparation • Expand access to and expedite clinical trials

Chapter 10: Advanced Health IT Strategies for Medical Practices

RPM and RTM further extend the capabilities of telemedicine by enabling continuous monitoring of patients' health status outside traditional clinical settings. RPM involves the use of digital technologies to collect health data from patients in one location and electronically transmit it to healthcare providers in a different location for assessment and recommendations. RTM, on the other hand, focuses on monitoring therapeutic outcomes and adherence to treatment plans, providing valuable insights into patients' responses to prescribed therapies.

These technologies are particularly beneficial for managing chronic conditions such as diabetes, hypertension, and heart disease, where regular monitoring is essential for effective disease management. By leveraging RPM and RTM, healthcare providers can detect early signs of deterioration, intervene promptly, and tailor treatment plans to individual patient needs, ultimately leading to improved health outcomes and reduced healthcare costs.

Strategies for Integrating Telemedicine

Integrating telemedicine into medical practices requires a strategic approach to ensure seamless adoption and optimal utilization. Before implementing telemedicine, it is crucial to assess the organization's readiness in terms of technology infrastructure, staff training and workflow integration. This includes evaluating existing IT systems, ensuring robust internet connectivity and identifying potential gaps that need to be addressed. Making sure that the provider has good lighting, can be seen on camera, has a microphone and also doesn't have any visible PHI in the camera's view are all also important parts to making telehealth successful. It is also helpful to have a provider champion that will be the first to try and work out any kinks. Providers are busy so you want to make sure that when you implement a new system you do it with someone that will be patient and understand that it will be a process to get it right. Picking the right person to be the champion can help ensure success and rapid adoption by the rest of the team.

Selecting the Right Telemedicine Platform

Choosing a telemedicine platform that meets the specific needs of the practice and its patients is essential. Factors to consider include ease of use for both the patient and the provider, dependability, costs, interoperability with existing EHR systems, data security and compliance with regulatory requirements such as HIPAA.

Training and Education

Comprehensive training programs for healthcare providers and staff are vital to ensure they are comfortable and proficient with the telemedicine technology. This includes training on how to conduct virtual consultations, troubleshoot technical issues and maintain patient engagement during remote interactions. It is always a good idea to practice a televisit with a staff member before going live with a real patient.

Developing Telemedicine Protocols

Establishing clear protocols for telemedicine visits helps standardize the process and ensures consistency in care delivery. This includes guidelines for patient triage, documentation, billing, copay collection and follow-up care. Protocols should also address situations where in-person visits are necessary, like how often the patient needs to be seen in the office.

Patient Engagement and Education

Educating patients about the benefits of telemedicine and how to use the technology is crucial for successful adoption. Providing clear instructions, offering technical support, and addressing any concerns or barriers to access can enhance patient engagement and satisfaction.

Ensuring Data Security and Privacy

Maintaining the confidentiality and security of patient data is paramount in telemedicine. Implementing robust cybersecurity measures, encryption protocols, and access controls can help protect sensitive information and build patient trust. Work with the telehealth vendor to make sure these securities are in place and also remember to not have any PHI in view of the camera when the provider is on a televisit.

Exhibit 10.3 Telehealth Workflow Cycle[8]

1. BEFORE THE VISIT

Patient Engagement and Education:
- Identifying patients likely to need additional support and developing a plan to set them up for success
- Educating patients on the offering
- Setting expectations for use
- Educating on proper appointment standard

Scheduling Protocols:
- Identifying appropriate clinical use cases
- Determining when/how telehealth visits will fit into the schedule
- Updating the EHR scheduler
- Identifying triage questions for scheduling appointments
- Ensuring clinicians are only providing care in states where they are licensed
- Ensuring telehealth is covered in clinicians' liability insurance

2. DURING THE VISIT

- Handling patient intake, "rooming" patients
- Supporting patient and clinician troubleshooting
- Setting up the exam room
- Communicating with patients

3. AFTER THE VISIT

- Knowing codes available for telehealth
- Integrating CP* codes and appropriate modifiers into the EHR
- Sharing visit summary and follow-up care

Leveraging RPM Technologies for Improved Patient Outcomes

RPM technologies offer significant potential for enhancing patient outcomes by enabling continuous, real-time monitoring of health parameters and facilitating timely interventions. Below is a screen shot from VitalCare Family Practice in Richmond Virginia. They use RPM with a company called Brilliant Care. You can see that of the 128 patients enrolled, 69% of them have had their disease state fall into the "controlled" status.

Exhibit 10.4 Example of Remote Patient Monitoring from Brilliant Care App

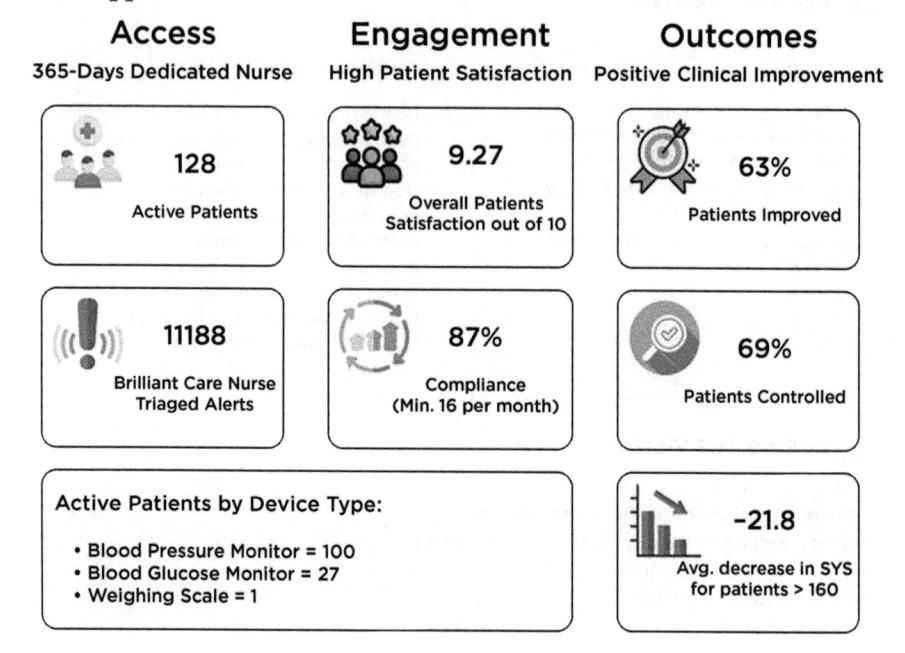

Access
365-Days Dedicated Nurse

- **128** Active Patients
- **11188** Brilliant Care Nurse Triaged Alerts

Active Patients by Device Type:
- Blood Pressure Monitor = 100
- Blood Glucose Monitor = 27
- Weighing Scale = 1

Engagement
High Patient Satisfaction

- **9.27** Overall Patients Satisfaction out of 10
- **87%** Compliance (Min. 16 per month)

Outcomes
Positive Clinical Improvement

- **63%** Patients Improved
- **69%** Patients Controlled
- **-21.8** Avg. decrease in SYS for patients > 160

Here are some keyways RPM technologies can be leveraged to improve patient outcomes:

Early Detection of Health Issues

RPM allows for the continuous collection of vital signs and other health metrics, enabling healthcare providers to detect early signs of deterioration or exacerbation of chronic conditions. Early detection can lead to prompt interventions, reducing the risk of complications and hospitalizations. RPM can also help with medication compliance. Many patients are better about taking their medicines when they know that their blood pressure is being monitored. They can see the results when they skip their medicine, which also increases compliance.

Chapter 10: Advanced Health IT Strategies for Medical Practices

Personalized Care Plans

By analyzing data collected through RPM, healthcare providers can gain valuable insights into patients' health trends and patterns. This information can be used to develop personalized care plans tailored to individual patient needs, improving the effectiveness of treatments and enhancing patient satisfaction.

For patients with chronic conditions, RPM provides a means of closely monitoring disease progression and treatment adherence. Regular monitoring can help healthcare providers adjust medications, recommend lifestyle changes, and provide timely support, ultimately leading to better disease control and quality of life.

RPM empowers patients to take an active role in managing their health by providing them with real-time feedback on their health status. Engaged patients are more likely to adhere to treatment plans, make informed decisions about their health, and adopt healthier behaviors.

Reduction in Healthcare Utilization

By enabling proactive management of health conditions, RPM can reduce the need for emergency room visits, hospital admissions and readmissions. This not only leads to cost savings for healthcare systems but also minimizes the burden on healthcare facilities and resources, making sure that patient care is happening at the right place at the right time.

Facilitating RTM

RTM focuses on monitoring patients' adherence to therapeutic regimens and tracking therapeutic outcomes. This is particularly useful for patients undergoing long-term treatments such as physical therapy or medication management, as it allows healthcare providers to assess the effectiveness of therapies and make necessary adjustments. We are starting to see RTM with things like devices that monitor medication adherence. For example, smart pill bottle tops know how many times they have been opened and medication dispensers can monitor medication adherence. At VitalCare Family Practice, they are doing new BioMech Gait and Balance RTM to help prevent falls in the elderly patient population. This Gait and

Balance device is the size of a thumb drive and can detect the position of the patient's pelvis as well as which foot hits the floor harder. It also measures the patients' balance so it can measure a patient's risk for falls.

Overcoming Barriers and Maximizing Benefits of Telemedicine

While the benefits of telemedicine and RPM are clear, there are several barriers to adoption that healthcare management professionals need to address to maximize the potential of these technologies. One of the primary barriers to telemedicine adoption is the complex and evolving regulatory landscape. Healthcare providers must navigate varying state and federal regulations, licensure requirements, and reimbursement policies. Staying informed about regulatory changes and advocating for supportive policies can help overcome these challenges. It is important to make sure that you or the RPM company that you are working with are compliant with the CMS regulations for billing RPM.

Technological Barriers

Ensuring access to reliable technology and internet connectivity is crucial for the success of telemedicine. Healthcare organizations should invest in robust telecommunication infrastructure and provide technical support to both providers and patients to address connectivity issues. By now, most patients have smart phones and that is all they need for telemedicine, but obviously some users are better with technology than others. We still hear providers say, "my patients are too old, they won't do telemedicine or RPM." However, more and more 80-year-olds have smartphones and are using technology more frequently. Also, some RPM providers provide devices that are cell enabled, so they don't even have to have a smart device to send the information back to the provider, so there are options for everyone.

Provider Resistance

Resistance to change among healthcare providers can hinder the adoption of telemedicine. Addressing concerns, providing adequate training, and highlighting the benefits of telemedicine for both providers and patients can help overcome this resistance. Also providing financial

Chapter 10: Advanced Health IT Strategies for Medical Practices

proformas can be a huge incentive for providers to adopt new technologies like this. In healthcare, we are not seeing pay increases from payers, but inflation is real, so adding revenue producing programs can help fight inflation. Integrating telemedicine into existing clinical workflows can be challenging. Healthcare organizations should focus on streamlining processes, ensuring interoperability with EHR systems, and minimizing administrative burdens to facilitate seamless integration. The AMA has a telehealth playbook that does a great job of outlining the steps:[9]

Measuring and Demonstrating Value

To sustain telemedicine initiatives, it is important to measure and demonstrate their value in terms of patient outcomes, cost savings, and patient satisfaction. Collecting and analyzing data on telemedicine usage and outcomes can provide valuable insights and support continuous improvement efforts.

Telemedicine, RPM, and RTM are transforming healthcare delivery by offering new opportunities for improving patient outcomes and enhancing access to care while optimizing healthcare management. By strategically integrating telemedicine into medical practices, leveraging RPM technologies and addressing barriers to adoption, healthcare management professionals can maximize the benefits of these innovations. As healthcare continues to evolve, embracing these elements will be essential for providing high-quality patient-centered care in the digital age.

10.5 Patient Engagement and Health Apps

In the digital age, patient engagement is increasingly being facilitated through digital platforms and mobile applications. These tools offer innovative ways to involve patients in their own health management, enhancing communication, adherence to treatment plans and overall health outcomes. A strategic approach is needed for engaging patients through digital platforms and mobile applications. Evaluating and integrating health apps into medical practices should be done in a way that promotes patient self-management and adherence while ensuring data security in patient engagement technologies.

Engaging Patients through Digital Platforms

Engaging patients effectively through digital platforms and mobile applications requires a multifaceted approach. The Office of the National Coordinator for Health Information (ONC) has a great health app playbook on patient engagement that provides some key strategies:[10]

User-Friendly Design and Communication Tools

Health apps must be intuitive and easy to navigate. A user-friendly interface encourages consistent use and engagement. Features such as simple navigation, clear instructions and visually appealing design are crucial. Having useful features such as prescription refill requests, messaging your provider, reviewing test results and scheduling appointments are great tools to have available in a health app. Direct communication features such as secure messaging with healthcare providers, requesting medication refills and viewing lab results can facilitate immediate support and guidance that enhances patient engagement.

Provider Recommendations

Practices can advertise their app all day long on their website, social media, and at the front desk, but the best way to encourage patients to use a health app or portal is by having the provider tell them that that is the preferred way to communicate with the practice. If the providers are not recommending and using the app, the patients won't either.

Evaluating and Integrating Health Apps into Medical Practices

Integrating health apps into medical practices requires careful evaluation and a structured approach. First, ensure that the health app can seamlessly integrate with existing EHR systems. This allows for smooth data exchange and continuity of care. Many EHRs have one app that you are required to use if you use their EHR, so you may not have much of a choice. However, this is an important decision when picking an EHR, because the app or patient portal can be one of the main ways you communicate with patients.

Provide training for healthcare providers on how to use the app and integrate it into patient care. Patients should also receive guidance on

Chapter 10: Advanced Health IT Strategies for Medical Practices

app usage to maximize its benefits. Include information about your app at check-in so that you can make sure patients get signed up. Also, make sure that your staff know how to use the app so they can help patients when they have issues. Regularly monitor app usage, patient feedback and health outcomes to assess the app's effectiveness. Continuous evaluation helps in making necessary adjustments and improvements. Below, you can see an example from VitalCare Family Practice on the Healow App analytics:

Exhibit 10.5 Healow App Analytics

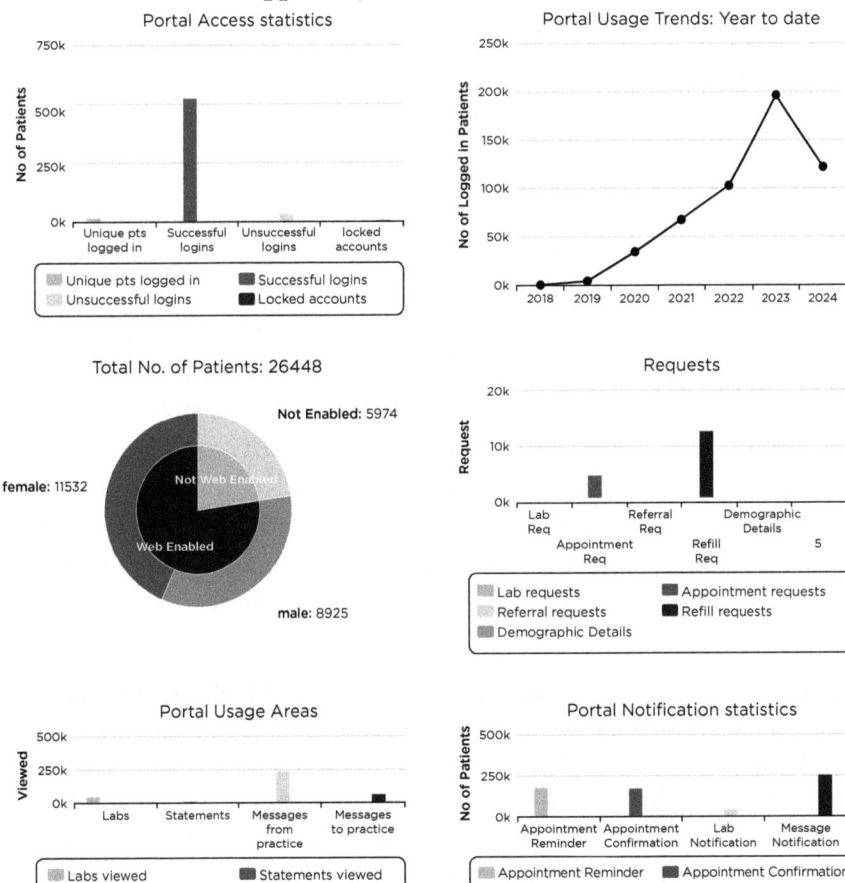

Ensuring Data Security in Patient Engagement Technologies

Ensuring the privacy and security of patient data is critical in the use of digital health tools. Health apps must comply with relevant regulations such as the HIPAA in the United States, which sets standards for the protection of health information. Make sure your app is HIPAA compliant and that your office uses it in a compliant manner. Conduct regular security audits and vulnerability assessments to identify and address potential security threats. Keeping software updated with the latest security patches is also essential. Implementing strong encryption protocols for data transmission and storage ensures that patient information remains confidential and secure from unauthorized access. Strict access controls ensure that only authorized personnel can access sensitive patient information. Multi-factor authentication (MFA) can add an additional layer of security.

Digital platforms and mobile applications are revolutionizing patient engagement by providing innovative tools for self-management, communication, and education. Successful integration of health apps into medical practices requires thorough evaluation, seamless EHR integration and continuous monitoring. Promoting patient self-management and adherence through features such as health tracking, reminders, and community support can significantly improve health outcomes. However, addressing privacy concerns and ensuring robust data security are paramount to maintaining patient trust and protecting sensitive health information. As technology continues to advance, the potential for digital tools to enhance patient engagement and improve healthcare delivery will only grow, making them indispensable in modern healthcare.

10.6 Cybersecurity and Data Privacy in Medical Practices

Cybersecurity and data privacy are paramount concerns for medical practices. As healthcare organizations increasingly rely on EHRs and other digital systems, they face a growing array of cybersecurity threats. Ensuring the security and privacy of patient data is not only a regulatory requirement, but also a critical component of maintaining patient trust and delivering high-quality care. Cybersecurity threats faced by medical practices require strategies for ensuring data security and privacy in EHR usage. By implementing robust security measures and training staff on cybersecurity awareness, your practice can keep in compliance with current data privacy regulations.

Cybersecurity Threats Faced by Medical Practices

Medical practices face numerous cybersecurity threats that can compromise patient data and disrupt healthcare delivery. Ransomware attacks involve malicious software that encrypts data and demands payment for its release. Ransomware can cripple medical practices by locking access to critical patient information and disrupting operations. A recent example of a ransomware attack was the Change Healthcare attack. UHG CEO Andrew Witty estimated that the data breach resulting from the Change Healthcare cyberattack will impact approximately one-third of Americans as the investigation continues.[11] This attack impacted physician practices all across the country. Even though it wasn't a direct attack on the practices, it took claims submission to a grinding halt and stopped income for practices. Change wound up paying $22 million dollars in bitcoin to the hackers. Below are other examples of cybersecurity threats that pose great risks to medical practices.

- **Phishing Scams:** Deceptive emails or messages designed to trick recipients into revealing sensitive information, such as login credentials. Phishing attacks are common in healthcare and can lead to unauthorized access to EHR systems or financial systems.
- **Insider Threats:** Risks posed by employees or contractors who have access to sensitive data. Insider threats can be intentional, such as theft of data, or unintentional, such as accidental data breaches due to negligence.
- **Advanced Persistent Threats (APTs):** Prolonged and targeted cyberattacks by sophisticated actors who aim to steal sensitive information over time. APTs often go undetected for long periods, causing significant damage.
- **Data Breaches:** Unauthorized access to patient data, which can result from weak security measures, vulnerabilities in software, or malicious attacks. Data breaches can lead to identity theft, financial loss and reputational damage.

Ensuring Data Security and Privacy in EHR Usage

Many medical practices work with IT professionals, however practice owners and administrators need to understand the basics to safeguard patient data within EHR systems. Medical practices must adopt comprehensive security strategies to reduce the risks of data breaches.

Training

The most important and least expensive way to avoid security threats is through end user training. Making sure that your own employees know how to recognize a phishing scam and understand how to report it are vital to data security. At the beginning of this chapter, we discussed how healthcare workers can lack technological knowledge and skills, therefore they are easy targets for phishing scams. Perform training and simulations to make sure your end users are wise and informed about these topics.

Encryption

Encrypting data both in transit and at rest ensures that patient information remains secure even if intercepted or accessed without authorization. Strong encryption protocols protect sensitive data from cyber threats. Many providers and staff use laptops and tablets for documentation. They also carry these devices around, so they can easily be lost or stolen. Encryption can provide security even if a device is lost or stolen.

Access Controls

Implementing strict access controls limits who can view or modify patient data. Role-based access control (RBAC) ensures that only authorized personnel have access to specific information based on their job responsibilities. For example, does the front desk staff need to be able to access clinical notes and does the clinical staff need to be able to access billing information?

Regular Audits

Conducting regular security audits and assessments helps identify vulnerabilities and ensure compliance with security policies. Audits should include reviewing access logs, monitoring unusual activities and testing for potential weaknesses. Annual security audits are a requirement for MIPS, so most practices should be doing them, however doing the audit is only the first step—you also need to make sure you review the audit and address any concerns that it uncovers.

Secure Authentication

Using multi-factor authentication (MFA) adds an extra layer of security by requiring multiple forms of verification before granting access. MFA reduces the risk of unauthorized access due to stolen or compromised credentials. Most banks require this by now and most users are used to this, but it is still somewhat hit or miss in healthcare facilities as to if they are using MFA or not.

Implementing Robust Security Measures to Protect Patient Data

Effective cybersecurity requires a multi-layered approach to safeguard patient data. The ONC has a security risk assessment tool with key measures.[12]

Deploy firewalls and intrusion detection/prevention systems (IDS/IPS) to monitor and block unauthorized access attempts. These tools help detect and respond to suspicious activities in real-time. Next, ensure that all software, including EHR systems, is up-to-date with the latest security patches. Regular updates prevent exploitation of known vulnerabilities. Also maintain regular backups of patient data and have a disaster recovery plan in place. Backups should be stored securely and tested periodically to ensure data can be restored in case of an incident. Lastly, protect devices such as computers, tablets and smartphones that access patient data. Endpoint security solutions include antivirus software, endpoint encryption and mobile device management (MDM) systems.

Complying with Data Privacy Regulations and Ensuring Ethical Data Use

Compliance with data privacy regulations is essential for protecting patient information and avoiding legal penalties:

- **HIPAA Compliance:** In the United States, the Health Insurance Portability and Accountability Act (HIPAA) sets national standards for the protection of health information. Medical practices must implement administrative, physical and technical safeguards to comply with HIPAA requirements.
- **Ethical Data Use:** Ensuring that patient data is used ethically involves obtaining informed consent for data collection and usage, maintaining transparency about data practices, and respecting patient privacy rights.
- **Data Minimization:** Collecting only the data necessary for specific purposes and retaining it only as long as needed. Data minimization reduces the risk of exposure and ensures compliance with privacy principles.

Training Staff on Cybersecurity Awareness and Best Practices

Not putting your user ID and password on a sticky note on your desk is a great place to start, but staff training is a critical component of a robust cybersecurity strategy. Regularly educate staff on cybersecurity threats, safe online practices and the importance of data protection. Training should cover recognizing phishing attempts, proper password management and reporting suspicious activities. Put that training into practice by conducting regular drills to prepare staff for potential cybersecurity incidents. Drills help ensure that everyone knows their role and can respond effectively to minimize damage and that the office can continue to function. This topic could be a whole book by itself, but the first things to think about for a medical practice is how will you know who is coming in tomorrow and how can you document for the patients that are here today? At a minimum, have answers to those questions in the event that your EHR system goes down.

Most importantly, foster a culture of security within the organization where all employees understand their responsibility in protecting patient data. Always encourage open communication about security concerns and promoting best practices. Making sure that staff feels safe to report when they have potentially had a security breach is crucial. If they feel

Chapter 10: Advanced Health IT Strategies for Medical Practices

like they will be reprimanded or fired for reporting an incident, they will likely hesitate to report such issues..

Cybersecurity and data privacy are critical components of modern medical practices. Understanding the threats, implementing robust security measures and complying with regulations are essential steps in safeguarding patient data. Additionally, training staff on cybersecurity awareness and best practices ensures a proactive approach to data protection. As cyber threats continue to evolve, medical practices must remain vigilant and adaptive to ensure the security and privacy of patient information, ultimately fostering trust and improving the quality of care.

10.7 Future Outlook

The future of health IT in medical practices looks promising as technological advancements continue to evolve. Several key trends and developments are expected to shape the landscape in the coming years. AI and machine learning are set to play a significant role in healthcare. These technologies can enhance diagnostic accuracy, personalize treatment plans and streamline administrative processes. For instance, AI-driven predictive analytics can help identify at-risk patients and suggest preventive measures, thereby improving health outcomes. Efforts to improve interoperability between different health IT systems will also continue to gain momentum. Standardized data exchange formats and protocols will facilitate seamless communication between healthcare providers, enhancing care coordination and patient safety. Additionally, advancements in blockchain technology could offer secure and transparent ways to manage health data.

The adoption of telehealth and remote patient monitoring will likely expand, driven by patient demand and the need for cost-effective healthcare solutions. These technologies will enable continuous patient engagement and real-time health monitoring, particularly for managing chronic conditions. The integration of wearable devices and mobile health apps will further support this trend. Digital health tools will continue to empower patients, giving them greater control over their health information and care decisions. Enhanced patient portals, mobile health apps, and personalized health interventions will foster patient engagement and improve adherence to treatment plans. As the reliance on digital health tools increases, so will the importance of robust cybersecurity measures. Medical practices will need to invest in advanced security technologies and foster a culture of cybersecurity awareness among staff. Ensuring compliance with evolving regulations and protecting patient data will remain a top priority.

The integration of advanced health IT strategies is essential for modern medical practices to thrive in an increasingly digital healthcare environment. By staying abreast of technological advancements and adopting a strategic approach to implementation, medical practices can overcome challenges and leverage health IT to deliver high-quality, efficient and patient-centered care. The future holds immense potential for health IT to revolutionize healthcare, making it more accessible, effective and sustainable for all.

10.8 Practice in Action

A residential services and support organization with more than 300 locations and a mission to provide exceptional community-based services that promote independent living and quality of life for individuals with special needs called upon the Change Healthcare Consulting team for a HIPAA Privacy and Security Assessment.[13] In addition, the client had a desire to map the HIPAA Security controls to the National Institute of Standards and Technology (NIST) Controls 800.53, version 4. The client had an impending audit and wanted to ensure compliance across the board adopting NIST as their cybersecurity framework. The client wanted the Change Healthcare team to assess and remediate their Privacy and Security program including, but not limited to, creating a set of Privacy and Security Policies and Procedures and conducting a high-level risk assessment. The Consulting team had a 4-month timeline to assess the client's current state and remediate the program.

The organization faced multiple challenges in their endeavor to maintain HIPAA Privacy and Security compliance. One critical challenge is the client's small size and heavy regulation requirements. Despite being a smaller organization, they faced the same policy and procedure requirements as a large company, yet with fewer resources. Another key challenge for the client was that, as a lean organization, they did not have the subject matter experts readily available to address their cyber security and privacy regulatory requirements. These gaps made it difficult to properly scope the engagement as the client was not entirely sure what they needed.

The primary goal for the Consulting team was to develop a scope and advise on that plan to ensure the client would pass the audit, but more importantly to reduce their security risk to an acceptable level for the organization. As a result, the Consulting team was able to conduct an initial assessment to identify deficiencies in their security program related to the HIPAA Privacy and Security Rule. To remediate, the Consulting team educated the staff on current rules and regulations through the development of a security training program and to understand their risks to be better prepared for future assessments. In addition, 32 privacy and 36 security policies and procedures were developed and delivered to the client.

The Consulting team was able to close out the project by leaving the client in a successful position, enabling them to pass audit and regulation checks in the future. The team carefully organized and structured the policies and procedures for easy review and ensured all staff was refreshed to maintain the new protocols moving forward.

10.9 Summary

The integration of health IT in medical practices is a transformative journey that promises substantial improvements in healthcare delivery. As explored in this chapter, health IT encompasses a wide array of tools and strategies—from EHRs and telemedicine to HIE and RPM. These technologies enhance operational efficiency, improve patient outcomes and support informed decision-making. However, the path to successful implementation is fraught with challenges ranging from high costs and interoperability issues to data security concerns.

Addressing these challenges requires a proactive and strategic approach. Effective training for healthcare providers combined with robust security measures and continuous evaluation are critical for optimizing the use of health IT. By leveraging advanced strategies and embracing innovative solutions, medical practices can overcome obstacles and fully harness the benefits of the most advanced healthcare tools. Furthermore, failure to advance and adopt new technology can cause practices to fall behind, leading to the inability to recruit new providers and staff.

Key takeaways from this chapter include:

- We examined the myriad ways in which health IT enhances the efficiency and effectiveness of medical practices. From digitizing patient records to enabling remote consultations, we highlight the tangible benefits that health IT brings to both healthcare providers and patients.
- Recognizing the obstacles that medical practices face in adopting health IT, we analyzed common challenges such as interoperability, data security, and regulatory compliance. By understanding these challenges, we can develop proactive strategies to address them effectively.
- Building upon foundational knowledge, we presented advanced strategies tailored to the unique needs of medical practices. From leveraging health analytics for predictive modeling to implementing interoperable systems, we offered practical insights to optimize the utilization of advanced healthcare technologies.
- Sustainable integration of health IT requires ongoing evaluation, adaptation and optimization. We discussed strategies for long-term sustainability along with financial implications, staff training, performance monitoring and continuous quality improvement initiatives.

The next and final chapter will cover the importance of effective risk management and compliance within a modern healthcare setting.

Chapter 10: Advanced Health IT Strategies for Medical Practices

Notes

1. MGMA. https://www.mgma.com/mgma-stats/measuring-the-rising-costs-of-health-it-compliance-in-medical-groups
2. MGMA. https://www.mgma.com/podcasts/executive-session-should-your-ehr-system-stay-or-should-it-go-
3. MGMA. https://www.mgma.com/mgma-stat/ehr-usability-patient-communications-billing-outrank-ai-as-top-tech-priorities
4. MGMA. https://www.mgma.com/articles/its-time-to-plan-the-funeral-for-fax-in-healthcare
5. MGMA. https://www.mgma.com/articles/navigating-the-constantly-evolving-cybersecurity-threat-landscape
6. MGMA. https://www.mgma.com/articles/release-of-information-what-you-dont-know-can-cost-you
7. AMA. https://www.ama-assn.org/system/files/ama-telehealth-playbook.pdf
8. AMA. https://www.ama-assn.org/system/files/ama-telehealth-playbook.pdf
9. AMA. https://www.ama-assn.org/system/files/ama-telehealth-playbook.pdf
10. HealthIT.gov. https://www.healthit.gov/playbook/pe/
11. Health IT Security. https://healthitsecurity.com/news/change-healthcare-disconnects-system-amid-cyberattack
12. HealthIT.gov. https://www.healthit.gov/topic/privacy-security-and-hipaa/security-risk-assessment-tool
13. Change Healthcare. https://www.changehealthcare.com/insights/hipaa-privacy-security-program-assessment

Chapter 11

Managing Risk and Compliance in a Medical Practice

By: Cristy Good,
MPH, MBA, CPC, CMPE

11.1 Introduction

Medical practices face several challenges and uncertainties that can impact their ability to provide quality care while maintaining operational efficiency and compliance. From clinical errors and patient safety concerns to regulatory changes and financial risks, the healthcare environment is full of potential risks for both patients and providers. Effective risk management strategies are important for medical practices not only to mitigate potential threats and safeguard reputation, but also to ensure patient safety while sustaining success.

This chapter reviews the critical importance of risk management in medical practices, examining the various types of risk that practices encounter and the proactive measures they can undertake to identify, assess and mitigate them. By understanding the significance of risk management and adopting a comprehensive approach to mitigation, medical practices can enhance patient safety, protect reputations and foster a culture of continuous improvement. This chapter aims to equip practice leaders and healthcare professionals with the knowledge and tools necessary to navigate the complexities of risk management and support their practices against emerging challenges.

11.2 Identifying and Assessing Risks

Ensuring the safety and financial stability of healthcare operations requires efficient risk management from leadership and staff. *The New England Journal of Medicine* defines risk management in the context of healthcare as the clinical and administrative systems, processes and reports employed to detect, monitor, assess, mitigate and prevent risks.[1] Medical practices encounter a broad spectrum of risks that can typically be categorized into four key areas: clinical, operational, financial and legal.

Clinical Risks

Clinical risks are directly related to patient care and outcomes. This includes both diagnostic and medication errors. Diagnostic errors may involve incorrect or delayed diagnosis, which can result in inappropriate treatment or delayed treatment for patients. These errors can have serious consequences and may lead to patient harm or even death. Medication errors can also occur at various stages, such as prescribing, dispensing, administering or monitoring medications. These errors can lead to adverse events and patient harm.

There is also the issue of overall patient safety to consider. Healthcare-associated infections (HAIs) that patients acquire while receiving treatment, such as surgical site infections or bloodstream infections may occur due to hand hygiene, sterilization, and disinfection protocols not being followed correctly. Falls are another safety risk for patients, especially the elderly or those with mobility issues. Implementing fall prevention strategies such as regular assessments of patient space, environmental modifications, and patient education can help reduce the risk of falls and related injuries. Surgical procedures carry risks and complications such as infections, bleeding and anesthesia-related concerns. To minimize risk, it is important to conduct preoperative assessments, follow surgical

Chapter 11: Managing Risk and Compliance in a Medical Practice

safety protocols and make sure postoperative care is communicated and followed. Malfunctioning medical devices also carries the risk of harming patients. Regular maintenance, equipment checks and prompt reporting of any issues are necessary for safety.

Below are some other common issues associated with clinical risks.

- **Communication Breakdown:** Communication failure between healthcare providers, patients, and other stakeholders can lead to misunderstandings, delays in care and errors in treatment. Effective communication is essential for patient safety and care coordination.
- **Documentation Errors:** Incomplete or inaccurate documentation can lead to errors in patient care, miscommunication, and legal issues. Be sure to keep medical records accurate and comprehensive to ensure continuity of care and patient safety.
- **Staffing and Workload Issues:** Inadequate staffing levels, excessive workloads, and burnout can contribute to errors and compromise patient safety.
- **Patient Confidentiality and Data Security:** Protecting patient information and maintaining data security is not only important, it's also mandated. Privacy policies and secure EHR systems are crucial, but make sure that all staff and patients are trained in data protection as well.

Operational Risks

Operational risks pertain to the day-to-day functioning of the medical practice.[2] These risks lead to the potential for losses or damage related to failures or inadequacies in internal processes, systems, people, or external events. Many of these can overlap with clinical risks as well.

One of the biggest operational risks involve staffing shortages. Having an insufficient number of healthcare professionals combined with poor workforce planning and ineffective management can negatively affect patient care and overall practice efficiency. Workflow inefficiencies often lead to delays resulting from reduced productivity and increased error rates. Clear communication channels emphasizing standardized protocols through regular team meetings are important to ensure smooth operations and patient safety. Supply chain disruptions can create shortages of necessary medical supplies and equipment, which can disrupt patient care, compromise quality and safety, and increase costs to an organization. Having contingency plans such as working with alternative suppliers can help minimize such risks.

Operational risks can also result from breakdowns in EHR systems or other critical IT infrastructure. Outdated technology systems paired with inadequate maintenance can affect patient safety. Data breaches can compromise patient privacy, leading to financial loss and damage to the organization's reputation. According to a February 2022 MGMA Stat poll, 16% of U.S. medical practices experienced a cyber-attack or ransomware attack in 2021.[3] Remember that non-compliance with healthcare regulations, licensing requirements and accreditation standards can result in legal penalties, loss of reputation, and even potential closure of the practice. As previously discussed, HIPAA and EMTALA violations carry fines, so it's important to have strong cybersecurity measures in place to protect information and make sure staff are trained. Contingency plans should also be in place in case systems go down.

Financial Risks

Financial risks can significantly impact the economic health of a medical practice. One major example involves issues with revenue cycle management. Problems with billing, coding and collections can affect cash flow. As discussed in Chapter 8, benchmarking KPIs can help organizations monitor their RCM processes. Reimbursement changes also create financial risks. Healthcare payers—both government and private insurers—may reduce insurance reimbursement rates for various services while updating payer policies that can impact the revenue of medical practices. There's also the issue of rising supply and labor costs. Inflation and the high cost of goods can increase supply costs. An increase in the cost of labor, particularly contract labor, can also put financial pressure on practices. Many are facing challenges in accessing capital due to rising levels of debt, tight liquidity, declining margins and being drawn on credit. Without access to capital, medical practices may struggle to modernize their facilities and optimize EHR systems.

More patients are participating in flexible coverage options and may seek care outside traditional sources or may choose not to seek care at all due to costs of services. Other reasons patients may choose to go elsewhere may be due to ineffective patient retention strategies, provider retirements that have been on the increase, and lack of expertise especially in practices experiencing high staff turnover.

Legal Risks

Legal risks involve potential litigation and regulatory penalties. Lawsuits filed by patients for alleged negligence or harm can include misdiagnosis, surgical errors, medication errors or failure to obtain informed consent. Healthcare professionals can face personal liability for their actions or omissions in providing medical care. This includes allegations of negligence, errors in treatment or failure to meet professional standards of care. Conflicts arising from agreements with vendors, insurers or employees can also create legal risks for medical practices. Failure to fulfill contractual obligations or disputes over contract terms can result in legal actions and financial consequences.

Failure to adhere to healthcare laws and regulations, such as HIPAA and OSHA standards can lead to legal penalties and reputational damage. Failure to protect patient data can also lead to legal liabilities and regulatory penalties. Medical practices must also ensure compliance with employment labor laws such as minimum wage, fair hiring practices, proper employee classification and overtime regulations.

Establishing a Risk Management Framework Assessment

The first crucial step in developing effective risk management strategies is establishing a robust framework. This process involves identifying potential risks, evaluating their impact and developing strategies to mitigate them. Breaking down this process into five steps provides a roadmap to moving forward with risk management strategies.[4]

1. **Risk Identification:** Begin by identifying all potential risks across the clinical, operational, financial and legal domains. Risk may include adverse events such as medical errors, security breaches, regulatory violations and operational disruptions. Identifying such risks can be achieved through various methods, including:
    - **Brainstorming Sessions:** Engaging staff members and stakeholders at all levels to discuss potential risks.
    - **Incident Reporting:** Reviewing past incidents and near-misses to identify recurring risks.
    - **Process Mapping:** Analyzing workflows to identify steps where errors or failures could occur.
    - **Regulatory Audits:** Examining compliance with regulations to uncover potential legal risks.
2. **Risk Analysis:** Once risks are identified, analyze them to understand their potential impact and likelihood.
    - **Severity Assessment:** Evaluating the potential consequences of each risk, such as harm to patients, financial loss, or legal repercussions.
    - **Likelihood Assessment:** Estimating the probability of each risk occurring based on historical data and expert judgment.
3. **Risk Evaluation:** Prioritize the identified risks by combining their severity and likelihood assessments. This helps the team focus on the most critical risks that require immediate attention.

4. **Risk Mitigation/Treatment Strategies:** Mitigation strategies may include implementing safety protocols, improving clinical processes, updating staff training and education, implementing quality improvement initiatives, and strengthening information security measures.

5. **Monitoring and Review:** Risk assessment is an ongoing process, so it is important that healthcare organizations monitor key risk indicators, track the implementation of risk mitigation measures, and review risk assessment findings periodically to identify possible emerging risks and opportunities for improvement.

Exhibit 11.1 Five Steps of Risk Management

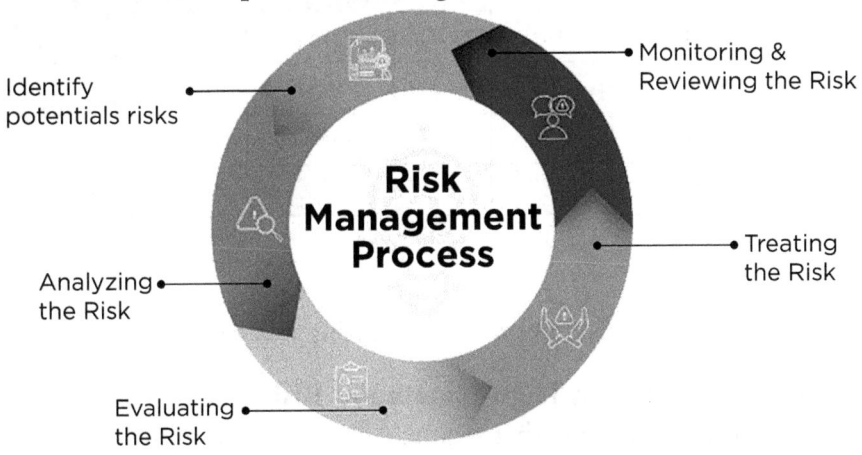

- Identify potentials risks
- Analyzing the Risk
- Evaluating the Risk
- Treating the Risk
- Monitoring & Reviewing the Risk

Risk Management Process

Documentation in each of these steps may include risk assessment reports, risk registers, action plans and incident reports. Findings and mitigation strategies should be documented and reported within the organization to ensure transparency, accountability and regulatory compliance.

257

Prioritizing Risks

Once the process is established, prioritize risks based on their potential impact and the probability of their occurrence. This prioritization enables medical practices to allocate resources efficiently and address the most significant risks first. A risk matrix is a useful tool for plotting the severity of risks on one axis and their likelihood on the other, creating a visual representation of risk levels.[5]

Exhibit 11.2 Risk Matrix Example

Impact — How severe would the outcomes be if the risk occurred?

Probability — What is the probability the risk will happen?

	Insignificant 1	Minor 2	Significant 3	Major 4	Severe 5
5 Almost Certain	Medium 5	High 10	Very high 15	Extreme 20	Extreme 25
4 Likely	Medium 4	Medium 8	High 12	Very high 16	Extreme 20
3 Moderate	Low 3	Medium 6	Medium 9	High 12	Very high 15
2 Unlikely	Very low 2	Low 4	Medium 6	Medium 8	High 10
1 Rare	Very low 1	Very low 2	Low 3	Medium 4	Medium 5

Safety Culture

Below is a breakdown of each intersecting risk level:

- **High-Severity, High-Likelihood Risks:** These are the most critical risks that require immediate and robust mitigation strategies.
- **High-Severity, Low-Likelihood Risks:** Although these risks are less likely to occur, their potential impact warrants careful monitoring and contingency planning.
- **Low-Severity, High-Likelihood Risks:** These risks occur frequently but have a lower impact. They require routine management and process improvements.
- **Low-Severity, Low-Likelihood Risks:** These are the least critical risks and may be addressed with standard operating procedures.

Other Tools and Frameworks for Risk Analysis

Various tools and frameworks can help identify, assess and manage risks systematically. One effective tool—often associated with Lean Six Sigma philosophies of reducing waste and promoting continuous improvement—is a SWOT Analysis. This tool helps identify strengths, weaknesses, opportunities and threats related to risk management.

- **Strengths and Weaknesses:** Internal factors that affect the practice's ability to manage risks
- **Opportunities and Threats:** External factors that could influence risk levels

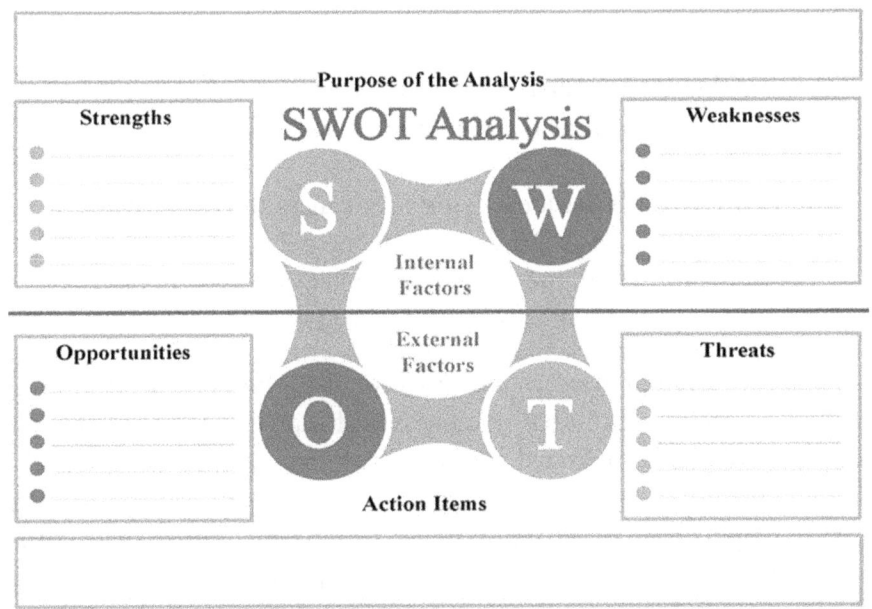

Exhibit 11.3 SWOT Analysis

Another effective risk analysis tool is a Failure Mode and Effect Analysis (FMEA). This is a systematic method for evaluating processes to identify where and how they might fail and assessing the relative impact of different failures. Usually, a nine-column table is used to help with this analysis. This type of analysis can be time and resource intensive.[6]

- **Failure Modes:** Potential ways in which a process could fail
- **Effects Analysis:** The consequences of these failures

Exhibit 11.4 FMEA Table

Steps in the Process	Failure Mode	Failure Causes	Failure Effects	Likelihood of Occurrence (1-10)	Likelihood of Detection (1-10)	Severity (1-10)	Risk Profile Number (RPN)	Actions to Reduce Occurrence of Failure
1								
2								
3								

A Root Cause Analysis (RCA) is a method used to identify the underlying causes of an incident or risk. This tool includes the following elements:[7]

- **Problem Identification:** Defining the risk or incident
- **Data Collection:** Gathering relevant information and evidence
- **Cause Analysis:** Identifying root causes through techniques like the "5 Whys" or fishbone diagrams
- **Solution Implementation:** Developing and implementing strategies to address root causes

Two commonly used frameworks for risk management provide a structured approach to identify, assess and manage risks. Healthcare organizations have integrated enterprise risk management (ERM) and/or ISO 31000 into their strategic planning processes. By considering risks and opportunities during strategic decision-making, organizations can align their resources and objectives for a proactive and risk-focused approach.

Enterprise Risk Management (ERM)

ERM is a broader approach to risk management that integrates risk assessment and mitigation across all areas of medical practice and organization. One way to define it is a set of actions or policies that aim at value protection and risk prevention for the organization by minimizing malpractices.[8] It includes conducting risk assessment surveys, formal risk reporting, and patient safety evaluation systems to create a culture of prevention and risk awareness throughout. Traditional ERM and value-based ERM frameworks are two healthcare risk management approaches. While both aim to identify and manage risks, they have key differences.

Traditional ERM Frameworks:

- Focus on reactive strategies for mitigating risks. They primarily aim to protect value by identifying and addressing risks that could negatively impact the organization.
- Often operate in silos, with different departments or units managing risks independently which may lead to fragmented risk management efforts and a lack of coordination.
- Typically focus on insurable risks, such as medical malpractice, general liability, and property loss and may not consider nonclinical risks or lost opportunities.
- May not fully integrate clinical and financial risks which could lead to not accounting for the relationship between clinical outcomes and financial performance.

Value-Based ERM Frameworks:

- Take a proactive approach to risk management. They not only aim to protect value but also focus on creating, recognizing and enhancing value.
- Take a holistic view of risks, considering both clinical and financial aspects.
- Address a wide range of risks, including environmental, competitive, strategic, financial, regulatory, operational, technological and reputational risks. They consider risks beyond traditional insurable categories.
- Are designed to align with value-based care models and payment systems.

Exhibit 11.5 Traditional ERM vs Value-Based ERM

COMPARISON OF TRADITIONAL AND VALUE-BASED HEALTHCARE ENTERPRISE RISK MANAGEMENT (ERM) FRAMEWORKS

Traditional ERM Framework
Risk Domains

- Operational
- Clinical/Patient Safety
- Strategic
- Financial
- Human Capital
- Legal/Regulatory
- Technology
- Hazard

Value-Based ERM Framework
Risk and Opportunity Domains

- Clinical Performance
- Strategic
- Human Capital
- Legal/Regulatory
- Technology
- Operational
- Financial

ISO 31000

ISO 31000 is an international standard for risk management that provides guidelines and principles for effective risk management practices.[9] It can be used by small and large organizations, helping them improve the identification of opportunities and threats and allocate resources for risk treatment. Utilizing ISO 31000 can help organizations achieve their objectives while effectively allocating and using resources for risk treatment. Additionally, it addresses operational continuity by providing a level of reassurance regarding economic resilience, professional reputation, and environmental and safety outcomes.

Identifying and analyzing risk in a healthcare setting involves understanding various risk types and prioritizing them effectively. Visualizing and addressing the most critical issues through various tools can be invaluable in systematically examining potential weaknesses and failures. Incorporating these methods into a robust framework ensures a comprehensive approach to mitigating risks and enhancing overall organizational resilience.

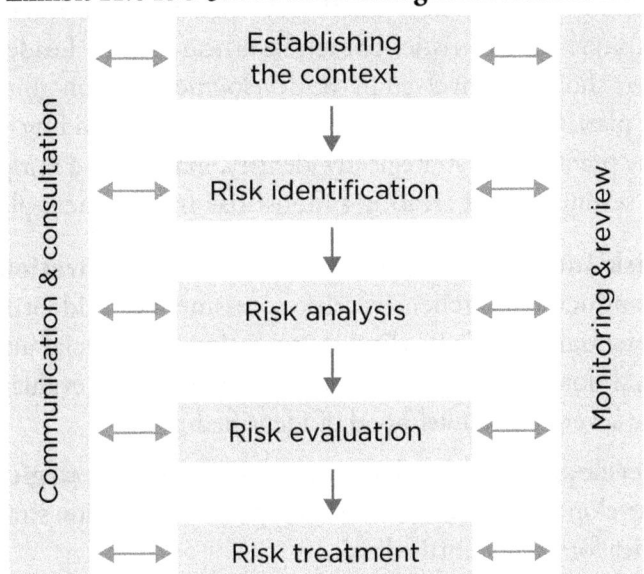

Exhibit 11.6 ISO 31000 Risk Management Framework

```
                    Establishing
                    the context
                         ↓
                   Risk identification
                         ↓
                    Risk analysis
                         ↓
                   Risk evaluation
                         ↓
                   Risk treatment
```
(Communication & consultation ← → | → ← Monitoring & review)

11.3 Developing Risk Management Strategies

A comprehensive risk management plan is the foundation of effective risk mitigation in healthcare. This plan should be tailored to the medical practice's specific needs and circumstances, considering its size, scope of services, patient population and unique risk profile. Once risks have been identified, assessed and prioritized, a comprehensive risk management plan should include:[9]

- **Risk Mitigation Strategies:** Specific actions to reduce the likelihood or impact of risks
- **Resource Allocation:** Assigning necessary resources, including staff, technology, and budget, to manage risks
- **Communication Plan:** Ensuring that all stakeholders are informed about risks and risk management strategies

- **Monitoring and Evaluation:** Regularly reviewing and updating the risk management plan to address new risks and changing circumstances

The format of a risk management plan can vary by organization and is contingent on the analysis of existing systems and historical data along with the unique characteristics of each healthcare entity. Leadership and stakeholders should be involved in the development and on-going evaluation of the plan. Once established, this plan will be the guiding document for how the practice will strategically identify, manage and mitigate risks. Below are seven steps for creating a robust risk management plan.

1. **Risk Identification, Assessment and Prioritization:** Conduct comprehensive risk assessments to identify potential hazards in clinical, operational, financial and legal domains. Utilize tools like risk matrices to evaluate the severity and likelihood of identified risks.

2. **Developing and Implementing Mitigation Strategies:** Develop a detailed plan outlining specific mitigation strategies for each identified risk.

    - **Administrative Controls:** Establish clear policies and procedures to guide staff behavior and decision-making processes. For example, strict protocols for medication administration should be implemented to prevent errors.
    - **Engineering Controls:** Modify the physical environment to eliminate or reduce hazards. This can include installing handrails, improving ventilation systems or using safety-engineered devices to prevent needlestick injuries.
    - **Personal Protective Equipment (PPE):** Provide necessary PPE to protect staff and patients from exposure to infectious agents or hazardous substances.

3. **Training and Education:** Conduct regular training sessions to ensure that all staff members know potential risks

and the measures in place to mitigate them. Incorporate simulation exercises to practice emergency responses and reinforce learning.

4. **Monitoring and Review:** Continuously monitor the effectiveness of risk mitigation measures through regular audits and feedback mechanisms. Review and update risk mitigation strategies as new risks emerge or existing ones evolve.

5. **Incidence Response:** Develop timely response protocols that call for immediate action. First, a root cause analysis will be conducted, and then the appropriate corrective actions will be implemented.

6. **Communication and Documentation:** Clearly communicate to all staff and include all stakeholders. Securely maintain and store all documentation for future reference.

7. **Evaluate and Improve:** Continuous process improvement involves a consistent stakeholder feedback loop.

Below is a sample outline that an organization can follow as it develops its risk management plan. While this Word document format is one of many templates that can be used, some use Excel to track the same information and add red/yellow/green to track progress.

I. Executive Summary

- **Introduction**: Brief overview of the risk management plan's purpose and scope.
- **Objectives**: Key goals and objectives of the risk management plan.
- **Scope**: Plan coverage, including departments, services, and activities.

II. Risk Management Governance

- **Risk Management Committee**: Formation, roles, and responsibilities.

- **Leadership and Accountability**: Roles of senior management in overseeing the plan.
- **Communication Strategy**: How risk management activities will be communicated within the organization.

III. Risk Identification

- **Types of Risks**: Clinical, operational, financial, legal, technological, environmental, etc.
- **Risk Assessment Tools**: Description of tools and techniques used to identify risks (e.g., SWOT analysis, risk assessments, audits).
- **Data Collection Methods**: Sources and methods for gathering relevant data.

IV. Risk Assessment and Analysis

- **Risk Assessment Framework**: Process for evaluating and prioritizing risks.
- **Risk Rating Criteria**: Criteria for determining the severity and likelihood of risks.
- **Risk Prioritization**: Process for ranking risks based on their potential impact and probability.

V. Risk Mitigation Strategies

- **Risk Mitigation Plan**: Strategies for reducing or eliminating identified risks.
- **Policies and Procedures**: Development and implementation of policies to mitigate risks.
- **Training and Education**: Programs to educate staff on risk awareness and mitigation techniques.

VI. Incident Response

- **Incident Response Plan**: Procedures for responding to and managing incidents.
- **Reporting Mechanisms**: Systems for reporting and documenting incidents.

Chapter 11: Managing Risk and Compliance in a Medical Practice

- **Root Cause Analysis**: Methodology for analyzing the underlying causes of incidents.

VII. Monitoring and Evaluation

- **Continuous Monitoring**: Processes for ongoing monitoring of risks and risk management activities.
- **Performance Metrics**: KPIs for measuring the effectiveness of risk management efforts.
- **Regular Audits and Reviews**: Scheduled audits and reviews to assess the risk management plan's performance.

VIII. Communication and Documentation

- **Internal Communication**: Strategies for communicating risk management policies and procedures to staff.
- **External Communication**: Procedures for communicating with external stakeholders about risk-related issues.
- **Documentation Standards**: Guidelines for documenting risk management activities and incidents.

IX. Compliance and Legal Considerations

- **Regulatory Compliance**: Ensuring adherence to relevant laws and regulations.
- **Legal Risk Management**: Strategies for managing legal risks and liabilities.
- **Patient Privacy and Confidentiality**: Measures to protect patient information and comply with privacy regulations (e.g., HIPAA).

X. Continuous Improvement

- **Feedback Mechanisms**: Processes for collecting and incorporating feedback from staff and stakeholders.
- **Lessons Learned**: Approaches for applying lessons learned from incidents and risk assessments.
- **Plan Updates**: Procedures for regularly updating the risk management plan based on new information and evolving risks.

XI. Appendices

- **Risk Assessment Templates**: Sample templates and forms used in risk assessments.
- **Incident Report Forms**: Standardized forms for reporting incidents.
- **Training Materials**: Resources and materials used for staff training on risk management.
- **Glossary of Terms**: Definitions of key terms and concepts used in the risk management plan.

XII. Approval and Sign-Off

- **Signatures**: Approval and sign-off from key stakeholders and leadership.

Establishing Policies, Procedures and Protocols to Mitigate Risks

Establishing robust policies, procedures and protocols can help healthcare organizations ensure consistent high-quality care while mitigating risks. These guidelines should be clear, comprehensive and regularly reviewed to reflect current best practices and regulatory requirements. Below are seven key areas for policies and procedures within a medical practice.[10]

1. Develop protocols for common clinical procedures and patient care activities. These should include guidelines for diagnosis, treatment, medication administration, infection control and fall prevention. Guidelines for reporting and investigating adverse events, near misses, and patient complaints are also important to identify areas of improvement and prevent future incidents.

2. Establish procedures for administrative tasks, including patient scheduling, record keeping and billing. Ensure that workflows are streamlined and that staff are trained to follow established protocols.

3. Develop policies and procedures for accurate and complete documentation of patient information (medical history,

treatment plans, informed consent, etc.). Implement protocols for maintaining and securing patient records and establish guidelines for record retention and disposal based on legal requirements.

4. Create emergency response plans for various scenarios, such as natural disasters, medical emergencies and security threats. Conduct regular drills to ensure that staff are prepared to respond effectively.

5. Develop policies and procedures to ensure compliance with applicable laws, regulations, and accreditation standards, such as HIPAA, EMTALA, and CMS Conditions of Participation.

6. Implement policies to protect patient data and ensure compliance with regulations like HIPAA. This includes guidelines for data access, storage, and transmission, as well as protocols for responding to data breaches.

7. Implement policies and procedures for ongoing quality assurance and performance improvement activities, including regular audits, data analysis, and performance monitoring. Develop protocols for identifying and addressing areas of improvement such as reducing medical errors, improving patient outcomes, and enhancing patient satisfaction.

Developing effective policies and procedures requires involving stakeholders, practicing clear communication, providing regular training and promoting continuous improvement. Engage staff at all levels as their input is invaluable in creating practical and effective guidelines. Ensure that policies and procedures are clearly communicated to all staff members by using multiple channels to disseminate information such as meetings, emails and intranet postings. Regular training ensures staff understand and adhere to established policies and procedures—this should include initial training for new employees and ongoing education for existing staff. Finally, policies and procedures should be regularly reviewed and updated to reflect changes in best practices, technology, and regulatory requirements. Then, solicit feedback from staff to identify areas for improvement.

Implementing Patient Safety Initiatives

Patient safety is among the most critical components of risk management in healthcare. The World Health Organization defines it as the absence of preventable harm to a patient and reduction of risk of unnecessary harm associated with health care to an acceptable minimum.[10] Implementing patient safety initiatives can significantly reduce the incidence of adverse events and improve overall quality of care. All staff should feel empowered to speak up about potential risks and errors, so it is important to encourage open communication and a non-punitive approach to error reporting. Some organizations have a phone number or an email set up through their compliance department for incident reporting. Additionally, many practices have a compliance officer as the main point of contact and who's responsible for ensuring staff follow policies and procedures.

Challenges in Adopting Patient Safety Practices

Adopting patient safety practices in healthcare settings can be challenging due to various factors. However, these challenges can be overcome with proper strategies and approaches. Healthcare organizations must first navigate a complex regulatory environment that is always changing. Compliance with various laws, regulations, standards and industry-specific guidelines requires keeping staff regularly updated on changes to help keep the organization out of legal issues.

Resistance to Change and Reporting

Just like any other organization, medical practices deal with resistance to change. This can be addressed by engaging healthcare professionals, administrators and staff in the decision-making process to ensure their buy-in and active participation in implementing patient safety practices. Educate healthcare professionals about the significance of patient safety and its impact on improving patient outcomes and reducing adverse events. Offer training programs and resources to help healthcare professionals understand any change in policy or procedure and why it is important. Also establish a culture that encourages reporting of errors without fear of punishment or blame. Be sure to focus on learning and improvement rather than individual culpability. Develop user-friendly incident reporting systems that capture and analyze data on errors and near misses, allowing for the identification of systemic issues and the implementation of targeted interventions.

Lack of Standardization and Training

With staff turnover constantly a challenge, time constraints and evolving best practices can make it increasingly difficult to ensure staff are trained on the most up-to-date information. Leadership must ensure that all staff are adequately educated and trained on risk mitigation measures and that each member has the necessary knowledge and skills to identify and address risks. Implement standardized protocols and best practices based on the latest research and evidence to ensure consistent high-quality care. Encourage healthcare professionals to stay updated with the latest patient safety practices through ongoing education, training and participation in quality improvement initiatives.

Interoperability and Data Security

Healthcare organizations handle a huge amount of sensitive patient data, making them potential targets of cyberattacks and data breaches. As previously discussed in Chapter 10, robust data security measures and training for all staff to protect patient privacy can significantly reduce such risks. Applying these strategies can help ensure seamless and safe information sharing and collaboration among different healthcare providers and systems. Other challenges such as incompatible EHR systems and data silos can hinder effective risk mitigation. Healthcare organizations must proactively address interoperability challenges to facilitate timely and accurate information exchange. As technology evolves, healthcare organizations are still trying to figure out how to integrate AI while implementing safeguards to prevent large language models (LLMs) from being misused to generate health misinformation. Organizations must also evaluate AI's transparency with risk mitigation processes and any vulnerabilities.

Balancing Patient Care and Risk Management with Limited Resources

Healthcare organizations must balance providing high-quality patient care and implementing risk mitigation measures. The focus on patient care can sometimes overshadow risk management efforts, leading to potential risk identification and mitigation gaps. Allocating adequate financial, technological and human resources can help support the implementation of patient safety practices. Always prioritize patient safety in resource allocation decisions, emphasizing its long-term benefits in terms of improved patient outcomes and reduced healthcare costs.

Exhibit 11.7 Socio-technical Approach to Patient Safety[11]

Culture of Safety
Varies widely, evolves, is measurable and can be improved

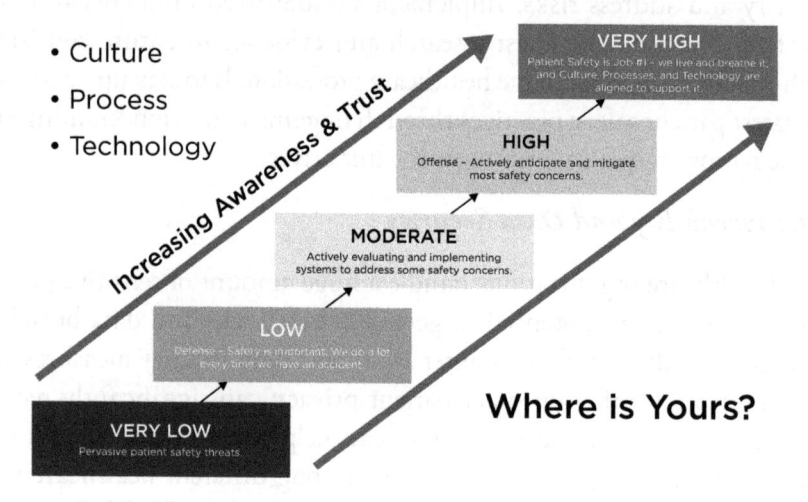

- Culture
- Process
- Technology

Increasing Awareness & Trust

VERY HIGH — Patient Safety is Job #1 - we live and breathe it, and Culture, Processes, and Technology are aligned to support it.

HIGH — Offense - Actively anticipate and mitigate most safety concerns.

MODERATE — Actively evaluating and implementing systems to address some safety concerns.

LOW — Defense - Safety is important. We do a lot every time we have an accident.

VERY LOW — Pervasive patient safety threats.

Where is Yours?

Key Patient Safety Initiatives

1. Establish protocols for medication management, including prescribing, dispensing and administration. Use technology, such as electronic prescribing and barcoding, to reduce the risk of medication errors.
2. Adhere to surgical safety checklists and review patient chart to prevent wrong-site surgery and surgical errors.

There should be protocols for surgical site infection prevention, including proper hand hygiene and sterile techniques.

3. Implement comprehensive infection control measures, including hand hygiene, sterilization of equipment and environmental cleaning. Develop protocols for early detection and management of healthcare-associated infections and protocols for isolation of infectious patients.

4. Implement systems for double-checking and verifying diagnostic tests and results. Promote open communication and collaboration among providers to discuss patient diagnosis and encourage ongoing training on diagnostic reasoning and clinical decision-making.

5. Conduct fall risk assessments for all patients and implement preventative measures. Patients and families should be educated on fall prevention strategies for those at risk. It is important for an organization to keep floors well maintained, have adequate lighting and handrails. Patients should be encouraged to report any falls to staff so that possible safety issues can be addressed and adverse events can be addressed.

6. Standardization of patient identification processes are important to prevent misidentification errors. Communication between patients and healthcare providers should be clear and understandable and a practice may need to seek interpretive services if needed to make sure patients understand their condition, treatment, and medications.

As the WHO states, investing in patient safety creates positive health outcomes, reduces costs related to patient harm, improves system efficiency and helps reassure communities by restoring their trust in healthcare systems.

Ensuring Compliance with Regulatory Requirements and Legal Considerations

Compliance with regulatory requirements and legal considerations can ensure that medical practices avoid significant penalties, legal liability and damage to the practice's reputation. Below are some key regulatory and legal requirements to consider.

1. **HIPAA Compliance:** Ensure that all patient data is protected in accordance with the Health Insurance Portability and Accountability Act (HIPAA). This includes implementing safeguards for data privacy and security, conducting regular risk assessments, and providing staff training.[12]

2. **OSHA Standards:** Comply with Occupational Safety and Health Administration (OSHA) standards to ensure a safe working environment for staff. This includes implementing safety protocols, providing necessary personal protective equipment (PPE), and conducting regular safety training.[13]

3. **CMS Regulations:** Adhere to Centers for Medicare & Medicaid Services (CMS) regulations regarding billing, coding, and reimbursement. Ensure that all claims are accurate and supported by appropriate documentation.[14]

4. **VAERS Reporting:** The Vaccine Adverse Event Reporting System (VAERS) is a national early warning system to detect possible safety problems in US-licensed vaccines. Healthcare professionals are required to report certain adverse events and vaccine manufacturers are required to report all adverse events that come to their attention.[15]

5. **State and Federal Laws:** Stay informed about state and local healthcare laws and regulations. This includes licensing requirements, reporting obligations and scope of practice regulations. The OIG (Office of Inspector General) creates compliance resources relevant to Federal health care laws and regulations.

Strategies for Ensuring Compliance

One of the first steps you can take toward compliance is appointing a compliance officer to oversee all aspects of regulatory compliance. This individual is typically responsible for developing and implementing compliance programs that include conducting audits and providing staff training. Developing comprehensive policies and procedures can ensure compliance with all relevant regulations. Regularly review and update these guidelines with the compliance officer to reflect changes in the regulatory landscape. From there, provide ongoing training and education to staff on regulatory requirements and best practices using a variety of training methods, such as workshops, online courses and simulation exercises. Be sure to conduct regular audits to assess compliance with regulatory requirements, then use audit findings to identify areas for improvement and implement corrective actions. Lastly, maintain thorough documentation of all compliance activities, including risk assessments, training sessions and audit findings. This documentation can serve as evidence of compliance in the event of an investigation or audit.

11.4 Incident Response

Responding promptly to incidents ensures patient safety and helps maintain the smooth operation of medical facilities. Risk mitigation in a healthcare setting involves a systematic approach to identifying potential hazards and implementing measures to reduce their likelihood and impact. This proactive strategy helps prevent adverse events and ensures compliance with regulatory standards.

Building a Culture of Safety and Encouraging Error Reporting

A culture of safety helps organizations reduce errors and enhance overall quality of care. Encouraging a non-punitive approach to error reporting empowers staff to identify and address issues before they escalate into serious incidents. This starts with the leaders. Leadership must demonstrate a strong commitment to safety by prioritizing it in all aspects of the organization's operations. Allocate resources for safety initiatives and ensure that safety policies are enforced consistently. Open communication is also key. Foster an environment where staff feel comfortable reporting errors and near-misses without fear of retribution. Implement anonymous reporting systems to encourage staff to report incidents they might otherwise hesitate to disclose. Once this is established, empower your staff through education and training. With ongoing training on best practices in patient safety and error prevention, educate staff on the importance of safety and the role they play in maintaining it. Recognize and reward staff who contribute to a safer workplace through innovative ideas or by reporting potential risks.

Establishing Incident Response Protocols and Procedures

When incidents occur, well-defined response protocols ensure they are managed effectively to minimize harm to patients and staff. As you develop your protocols, consider the key elements below.

- **Immediate Response:** Establish procedures for the immediate response to incidents, including medical intervention for affected individuals and containment of the situation. Designate response teams with specific roles and responsibilities.
- **Incident Reporting:** Implement a standardized process for reporting incidents, ensuring that all necessary information is captured accurately and promptly. Use electronic reporting systems to facilitate quick and efficient documentation.
- **Investigation and Documentation:** Conduct thorough investigations to determine the root causes of incidents. Document findings comprehensively to inform future prevention strategies.
- **Communication:** Communicate incident details to all relevant stakeholders including staff, patients and regulatory bodies as required. Maintain transparency while respecting patient and staff confidentiality.

Adopting a continuous improvement mindset helps organizations learn from incidents. Use insights gained from RCA to drive continuous improvement in safety practices and protocols, then share lessons learned across the organization to promote a culture of learning and prevention.

Incorporate findings from incident investigations into staff training programs, using case studies and real-life examples to illustrate the importance of adherence to safety protocols. Once this is set into place, policies and procedures should be regularly reviewed and updated based on the findings from incident investigations. Ensure that changes are communicated clearly to all staff members and integrated into practice.

11.5 Communication and Documentation

Communicating risks to staff, patients and stakeholders involves clear documentation of processes while educating staff on awareness and addressing patient concerns. This documentation should be both comprehensive and actionable, giving all organizational levels clear objectives and responsibilities. Several communication strategies are tailored for each level of engagement, from stakeholders to patients.

Communicating with Staff

- **Regular Meetings and Briefings:** Hold regular safety meetings and briefings to discuss potential risks, recent incidents, and preventive measures. Encourage open dialogue and feedback from staff to identify and address concerns promptly.
- **Use of Technology:** Implement digital platforms such as intranet portals, emails, and instant messaging to disseminate risk-related information quickly and efficiently. Utilize alert systems to notify staff immediately about urgent risks.
- **Visual Aids:** Use posters, infographics, and charts in common areas to highlight key risks and safety protocols. Ensure that visual aids are updated regularly to reflect current risks and mitigation strategies.

Communicating with Patients

- **Transparency and Honesty:** Be transparent with patients about potential risks associated with their care, including procedural risks, medication side effects and infection

control measures. Use clear, jargon-free language to ensure patients understand the information.
- **Patient Education Materials:** Provide educational materials such as brochures, pamphlets, and videos that explain common risks and the steps taken to mitigate them. Make these materials available in multiple languages and accessible formats to cater to diverse patient populations.

One-on-One Discussions: Encourage healthcare providers to discuss risks directly with patients during consultations. Allow patients to ask questions and express concerns, ensuring they feel heard and informed.

Communicating with Stakeholders

- **Regular Reports:** Provide regular risk management reports to stakeholders, including board members, regulatory bodies, and insurance companies. Include data on identified risks, mitigation efforts and outcomes.
- **Stakeholder Meetings:** Organize meetings with key stakeholders to discuss risk management strategies and outcomes. Seek input and collaboration from stakeholders to enhance risk management practices.

Ensuring Clear and Concise Documentation

Proper documentation not only ensures that risk management activities are traceable and transparent, but also promotes continuous improvement and accountability. Consider the key elements below when developing risk management documentation for your medical practice.

- **Standardized Forms and Templates:** Use standardized forms and templates for documenting risk assessments, incident reports, and mitigation plans. Ensure that these forms are easily accessible to all staff members.
- **Detailed Records:** Document all risk management activities in detail, including the nature of the risk, the assessment process, mitigation measures implemented, and outcomes.

Include dates, times and names of involved individuals for accurate record-keeping.
- **Confidentiality and Security:** Ensure that all documentation is kept confidential and secure, in compliance with data protection regulations such as HIPAA. Use encrypted digital systems and limit access to authorized personnel only.

Educating Staff on Risk Awareness

Educate staff about risks and their roles in proactive mitigation by developing comprehensive training programs that cover all aspects of risk management, including identification, assessment, mitigation and reporting. Using various training methods including lectures, workshops, simulations and e-learning modules, offer ongoing education and refresher courses to keep staff updated on new risks and evolving best practices. Encourage staff to participate in continuing education opportunities and professional development programs. Provide role-specific training that includes practical examples and case studies to ensure that each staff member understands the risks associated with their particular duties and responsibilities. By providing the knowledge and tools they need to identify and mitigate risks, this education can empower staff to take an active role in risk management with accountability.

Addressing Patient Concerns and Inquiries

Addressing patient concerns and risk inquiries effectively builds and maintains trust while ensuring patient satisfaction. Adopt a patient-centered approach to proactive communication, focusing on empathy and understanding. Listen actively to patient concerns and provide clear, accurate information in response. Establish dedicated resources, such as patient advocates or risk management officers, to address patient concerns and inquiries. Also be sure to provide contact information for these resources and encourage patients to reach out with questions. Follow up with patients who have expressed concerns to ensure their issues have been addressed to their full satisfaction, providing updates on any actions taken in response to their concerns. Implement feedback mechanisms such as surveys and suggestion boxes to gather patient input on risk management practices. Use feedback to identify areas for improvement and enhance the patient experience.

11.6 Monitoring and Evaluation

Effective monitoring and evaluation ensures that risk management efforts are continuously assessed, improved and aligned with organizational goals. To maintain a strong risk management program, healthcare organizations must establish a framework for continuous monitoring and evaluation. This involves regularly reviewing and assessing the effectiveness of risk management strategies and ensuring they address the evolving needs of the practice. This process can be broken down into three key elements.

- **Regular Audits and Reviews:** Conduct regular audits and reviews of risk management practices to ensure compliance with established protocols and policies. Schedule periodic evaluations to assess the effectiveness of risk mitigation measures and identify any gaps or weaknesses. Audits can be done both internally and by an external source.
- **Performance Metrics:** Develop and utilize performance metrics to measure the success of risk management strategies. Track key indicators such as incident rates, response times and patient safety outcomes. We mention a number of those metrics earlier in this chapter.
- **Stakeholder Involvement:** Involve key stakeholders—leadership, staff, patients and regulatory bodies—in the monitoring and evaluation process. Gather input from stakeholders to gain a comprehensive understanding of risk management performance.[16]

Collecting and Analyzing Data

By systematically gathering and examining data, healthcare organizations can make informed decisions and enhance their risk management efforts while identifying trends and areas for improvement. Utilize incident reporting systems to collect data on adverse events, near misses and other safety-related incidents. Encourage staff to report incidents promptly and accurately. Distribute surveys and feedback forms to staff and patients to gather insights on risk management practices and areas needing improvement. Ensure anonymity and confidentiality to encourage honest responses. Trend analysis and RCA are great tools for analyzing the data gathered from the methods above. Conduct trend analysis to identify patterns and recurring issues in risk management data. Use statistical methods to analyze data and determine the significance of identified trends. Perform root cause analysis on incidents and adverse events to uncover underlying factors contributing to risks. Develop targeted interventions based on the findings to prevent future occurrences.

Continuous improvement in risk management requires making necessary adjustments based on the findings from monitoring and evaluation efforts. This involves revising policies, procedures and practices to enhance the effectiveness of risk mitigation strategies. Review and update risk management policies regularly to reflect new insights and best practices. Ensure that revised policies are communicated to all staff and integrated into daily operations. Modify procedures and protocols to address identified gaps and weaknesses in risk management. Provide training and support to staff to facilitate the implementation of new procedures.

Incorporating Feedback and Lessons Learned

Incorporating feedback and lessons learned from monitoring and evaluation activities is essential for continuous improvement in healthcare risk management. By leveraging this information, organizations can enhance their risk management strategies and improve overall safety and quality of care. Actively seek and incorporate feedback from staff and patients on risk management practices. Use this feedback to identify areas for improvement and develop targeted interventions. Once the feedback is incorporated, conduct debriefing sessions following incidents to gather insights and lessons learned. Share these lessons with the wider organization to promote a culture of continuous learning and improvement. Integrate findings from monitoring and evaluation into quality improvement programs. Develop and implement initiatives aimed at addressing identified risks and enhancing patient safety. Provide ongoing education and training to staff on the importance of monitoring and evaluation in risk management. Encourage a proactive approach to identifying and mitigating risks. Some larger organizations have a continuous process improvement specialist or team to help with these processes as they arise.[17]

By implementing ongoing monitoring and evaluation processes, collecting and analyzing data, making necessary adjustments, and incorporating feedback and lessons learned, healthcare organizations can continuously improve their risk management strategies.

11.7 Practice in Action

Encompass Health faced significant challenges in establishing a comprehensive, HIPAA-compliant risk analysis process due to its vast and complex operations.[18] The organization operates 127 hospitals and 237 home health and hospice locations across 36 states and Puerto Rico, continuously expanding through acquisitions, which complicates the management of information assets and associated risks. The Chief Security Officer (CSO) at Encompass Health highlighted the inadequacies of previous risk analysis attempts that failed to adapt to the dynamic nature of the organization.

Upon joining Encompass Health, the CSO sought a solution that could provide an ongoing, adaptable risk management process aligned with OCR guidelines. Encompass Health partnered with Clearwater, a compliance and risk management provider in healthcare. This partnership introduced the organization to Clearwater's HIPAA Compliance and Cybersecurity BootCamp along with Clearwater's IRM|Pro software suite. Encompass Health was particularly interested in the IRM|Analysis module within the suite for its capability to implement and automate a continuous, OCR-compliant risk analysis process.

Clearwater's software-as-a-service (SaaS) model facilitated a quick deployment without upfront capital costs. Encompass Health opted for a comprehensive package that included software deployment, user training, and professional services to conduct the initial risk analysis. This approach minimized the impact on staff and ensured a swift, effective implementation.

Clearwater's team assisted Encompass Health by interviewing staff to identify and document information assets, organizing them to optimize the use of the software and the risk analysis process. This collaboration allowed Encompass Health to start the risk assessment process immediately, achieving in days what would have taken weeks independently. The entire process, from software deployment to the completion of the risk analysis, was finished in six months.

The partnership with Clearwater yielded significant benefits for Encompass Health:

- **Centralized Risk Data:** All information assets and their associated risks are now documented within Clearwater's IRM|Analysis system, simplifying risk management and reporting.
- **Real-Time Risk Analysis:** The new tools and processes enable real-time management of assets and risks, moving away from outdated, static risk analysis reports.
- **Adjustable Risk Tolerance:** The dashboard and embedded reports in IRM|Analysis allow the security team to adjust risk tolerance thresholds, addressing lower risk items as higher risks are mitigated.
- **Easy Report Generation:** The built-in reporting features facilitate the generation of up-to-date risk analysis reports for various stakeholders, including executive leadership, the Board of Directors, insurance risk providers, OCR, and third-party auditors.
- **Increased Confidence in Findings:** Centralized and current risk information provides assurance that regulatory requirements and OCR guidelines are being met.

11.8 Summary

In healthcare, effective risk and compliance management are critical to ensuring patient safety, regulatory adherence, and organizational resilience. This chapter has outlined the critical components of a comprehensive risk management framework tailored for medical practices, emphasizing a proactive and systematic approach.

- We began by categorizing the diverse risks inherent in medical practice—clinical, operational, financial, and legal. Conducting thorough risk assessments allows organizations to identify potential hazards and prioritize them based on severity and likelihood, using robust tools and frameworks to guide the analysis.
- Building on the assessment phase, we explored how to create a risk management plan customized to the practice's specific needs. Establishing clear policies, procedures, and protocols is essential to mitigate identified risks. Implementing patient safety initiatives and ensuring compliance with regulatory requirements further strengthen these strategies.
- Mitigating risks involves deploying practical measures and controls, fostering a culture of safety, and encouraging transparent error reporting. Establishing detailed incident response protocols ensures prompt and effective action when issues arise. Conducting root cause analyses enables learning from incidents, driving continuous improvement.
- Effective communication and meticulous documentation are critical for transparent risk management. Ensuring that staff, patients, and stakeholders are well-informed about risks and mitigation efforts is vital. Educating staff on risk awareness and their roles fosters a collaborative environment where patient concerns are quickly addressed.
- The final component involves ongoing monitoring and evaluation of risk management strategies. Collecting and analyzing data to identify trends, making necessary adjustments, and incorporating feedback ensures that risk management processes remain effective and adaptive to changing conditions.

A holistic approach to risk and compliance management in healthcare not only safeguards patient welfare but also enhances the operational integrity and reputation of medical practices. By integrating these strategies, healthcare organizations can navigate the complexities of risk, fostering a safer and more efficient care environment.

Notes

1. NEJM. https://catalyst.nejm.org/doi/full/10.1056/CAT.18.0197
2. LinkedIn. https://www.linkedin.com/advice/1/what-best-practices-measuring-operational-risk-imwcc
3. MGMA Stat. https://www.mgma.com/mgma-stats/cyberattacks-ransomware-still-a-growing-threat-for-medical-practices
4. HCI. https://hci.care/managing-risks-in-health-and-social-care/
5. Safety Culture. https://safetyculture.com/topics/risk-assessment/5x5-risk-matrix/
6. UNC. https://www.med.unc.edu/ihqi/wp-content/uploads/sites/463/2022/02/QIToolkit_FailureModesandEffectsAnalysis-2.pdf
7. NIH. https://www.ncbi.nlm.nih.gov/books/NBK570638/
8. Langate. https://langate.com/healthcare-enterprise-risk-management/
9. ISO.org. https://www.iso.org/iso-31000-risk-management.html
10. WHO. https://www.who.int/news-room/fact-sheets/detail/patient-safety
11. Health Catalyst. https://www.healthcatalyst.com/insights/safety-culture-healthcare-7-step-framework
12. HHS.gov. https://www.hhs.gov/hipaa/for-professionals/compliance-enforcement/index.html
13. OSHA.gov. https://www.osha.gov/complianceassistance/quickstarts/general-industry
14. CMS.gov. https://www.cms.gov/marketplace/resources/regulations-guidance
15. HHS.gov. https://vaers.hhs.gov/about.html
16. NIH. https://www.ncbi.nlm.nih.gov/pmc/articles/PMC7122203/
17. EDC. https://www.edc.org/blog/building-continuous-improvement-team
18. Clearwater Security. https://clearwatersecurity.com/case-studies/encompass-health-automates-its-hipaa-compliant-risk-assessment-strengthens-security-risk-management/

Conclusion

A*dvanced Strategy for Medical Practice Leaders: Operations Management Edition* aims to equip healthcare leaders with the strategic insights and practical tools necessary to navigate medical practice operations with confidence and efficiency. We began by establishing the foundational elements of mission, vision, and values—core components that set the tone for your organization's culture and success, guiding every strategic decision. Understanding how to align these elements while engaging key stakeholders and maintaining consistency in operational excellence and quality improvement is crucial to ensure effective operations management in healthcare.

From there, we explore the administrative structures that underpin effective medical practice operations. From leadership's influence to organizational design, and the implementation of health information systems, this book elaborated on the critical aspects that ensure operational efficiency. Staffing and operations underscores the significance of optimizing staffing models and employing strategic recruitment and retention practices. As we looked forward to future trends in staffing, including predictive analytics, we learned of the growing importance of diversity, equity and inclusion in healthcare leadership to foster a supportive and sustainable workforce.

Understanding the nuances of employed physician models while exploring emerging models like telehealth can help long-term operational success. Navigating the various financial models and revenue cycle management techniques, this book highlighted the dynamics of traditional, value-based and population-based care models. Effective financial management not only involves budgeting and revenue cycle management, but it also takes strategic negotiation and effective payer contracting to ensure your practice's financial health. Informed decision-making in all aspects of healthcare requires careful data management. The utilization of data through benchmarking and KPIs is vital for continuous improvement and maintaining a competitive advantage.

Marketing also plays a critical role in the success of medical practices in a competitive and ever-evolving industry. From developing a robust marketing strategy to leveraging patient testimonials and online reviews, we examined the tools and techniques necessary for engaging healthcare marketing. Adapting to future trends and technological innovations also ensures continued patient engagement and practice growth. The transformative impact of electronic health records (EHR), telemedicine, and cybersecurity requires implementing these technologies effectively while ensuring data privacy and security. All of this is accomplished through a comprehensive framework for managing risk and compliance. Medical practices must be proactive in identifying and assessing various risks while developing mitigation strategies and fostering a culture of safety and compliance.

As you move forward, remember that operations management is an ongoing journey. The principles and strategies outlined in this book are designed to be adaptable and scalable, allowing you to continuously evolve and improve your practice. Embrace the challenges, leverage the tools provided and strive for excellence in every aspect of your operations.

Index

A
ACA. *See* Affordable Care Act
Administrative Burden, 137, 141
Administrative Structures, 21
    components and workflow, 24
    importance of, 22
    leadership approach, 23
    leadership influence, 23
    organizational design, 24
Affordable Care Act (ACA), 35
Aging Physician Workforce, 100
Alternative Payment Model, 144
Ambulatory Surgery Centers (ASCs)
    closings impacted by patient demand, 86
Anti-Discrimination Laws, 67
    Age Discrimination Employment Act (ADEA), 67
    Americans with Disabilities Act (ADA), 67
    gender and sex, 67
    race and color, 67
    religion, 67
    Title VII of Civil Rights Act, 67
Applicant Tracking System (ATS), 52
Application Programming Interface (API), 226
Artificial Intelligence (AI) Integration, 214
Artificial Intelligence (AI) Prompts, 214
ATS. *See* Applicant Tracking System
Automated Data Reporting, 159

Automation, 57
    appointment scheduling, 60
    artificial intelligence (AI), 60
    data security, 61
    diagnostic imaging analysis, 60
    human intervention mechanisms, 61
    inventory management, 60
    natural language processing (NLP), 61
    patient communication, 60
    pharmacy automation, 61
    phased implementation, 62
    predictive analytics, 61
    prescription refills, 60
    repetitive tasks, 60
    virtual health assistant, 60

B
Baby Boomers (1946-1964), 110
Behavioral or Situational Interviewing, 53
Benchmarking
    benefits, 173, 177
    concepts, 172
    documentation, 177
    history, 173
    national accreditation organizations, 183
Benchmarking 10-Step Process, 176
Benchmarking Technology
    financial benchmarking, 175

Benchmarking Terminology
    functional benchmarking, 175
    performance benchmarking, 175
    process benchmarking, 175
    product benchmarking, 175
Benchmarking Types
    competitive benchmarking, 174
    internal benchmarking, 174
    strategic benchmarking, 175
Beveridge Model
    United Kingdom model, 119
Brand Identity
    content marketing, 203
    effective website, 202
    mission and values, 199
    online presence, 201
    value proposition, 199
    visual identity, 199-200

C
Centers for Medicare & Medicaid Services (CMS), 274
Charting, 126
Claims Denial Management, 127
Claims Processing, 127
Cleveland Clinic, 3
Clinical Risks
    bloodstream infections, 252
    fall prevention, 252
    healthcare-associated infections (HAIs), 252
    surgical site infections, 252
CMS. *See* Centers for Medicare & Medicaid Services
Communications
    digital platforms, 277
    one-on-one consultations, 278
    patient education materials, 278
    staff meetings and briefing, 277
    stakeholder meetings, 278
    transparency, 277
    visual aids, 277
Compensation
    annual percentage changes, 88

Consistency in Cultivating Culture
    alignment of efforts, 6
    culture reinforcement, 6
    trust and predictability, 6
Consolidated Appropriations Act, 2023, 93
Content Marketing
    local search engine optimization (SEO), 205
    online advertising, 204
    social media platforms, 203
Contract and Amendments Review
    penalties, 152
    rates, 152
    term, 152
    termination, 152
Contract Negotiation
    communication plan, 147
    value proposition, 147
Contract Negotiation Language, 152
Contract Performance Comparison, 139
Contract Proposal Elements, 142
Contract Proposal Preparation, 145
Contracting Vehicles, 146
Cultivating Culture, 6
Culture of Accountability, 55
Culture of High-Quality Care, 15
    innovation, 16
    patient-centric approach, 15
    reviews and adjustments, 16
    set clear goals, 15
    utilize data, 15
Cybersecurity, 240
    intrusion detection/prevention systems (IDS/IPS), 243
    password management, 244
    security-risk assessment tools, 243
    staff training drills, 244
Cybersecurity Threats
    advanced persistent threat (APT), 241
    data breaches, 241
    insider threats, 241
    phishing scams, 241

Index

D
Data Privacy
  data minimization, 244
  ethical data use, 244
  HIPAA compliance, 244
  regulation compliance, 243
Data Security, 35, 61, 240
  access control limits, 242
  audits and assessments, 242
  encryption, 242
  multi-factor authentication (MFA), 243
Data Sources
  federal and state agencies, 165
  for-profit benchmarking companies, 166
  Medical Group Management Association (MGMA), 164
  national accreditation organizations, 166
  professional associations, 165
Data Standardization, 167
DEI. *See* Diversity, Equity, and Inclusion
Diagnostic Testing Verification, 273
Diversity, Equity, and Inclusion, 63
  leadership roles, 65
  promotion strategies, 64

E
EAP. *See* Employee Assistance Program
EHR. *See* Electronic Health Record
Electronic Health Record (EHR), 162, 221
  ambient-listening devices, 224
  data entry tools, 224
  enhancement requests, 223
  user interface training, 223
Emergency Response Plans, 269
Employed Physician Model, 78
  advantages, 79
  challenges, 80
  engagement and retention, 81
  independent practitioners, 78
  salaried employees, 78
Employee Assistance Program (EAP), 56
Employee Engagement Elements
  growth opportunity, 55
  hands-on management, 55
  meaningful work, 55
  positive work environment, 55
  trust in leadership, 55
Employee Engagement Strategies, 55
Employee Engagement Surveys, 54, 56
Engagement with Physicians, 82
  physician liaison programs, 82
  psychological safety, 82
  regular feedback sessions, 82
Engaging Your Healthcare Team, 14
  collaboration, 14
  communication, 14
  training and education, 14
Enterprise Risk Management (ERM), 260
Examine Workspace, 12

F
Failure Mode and Effect Analysis (FMEA)
  effects analysis, 260
  failure modes, 260
Fall Risk Management, 273
Family Medical Leave Act (FMLA), 66
Fee-for-Service Aggregate Equivalency, 142
Financial and Performance Data
  Electronic Health Record (EHR), 162
  employee payroll systems, 163
  financial statements, 160
  patient social media postings, 163
  patient surveys and feedback, 163
  Practice Management System (PMS), 162
  regulatory and compliance data, 163
Financial Indicators Related to Staffing, 42
  benefit cost-total salary ratio, 43
  labor cost per patient day, 42

291

overtime percentage, 43
staffing expense ratio, 42
Financial Management, 29
    accounts receivable, 31
    budgets and financial planning, 30
    cost optimization, 32
    revenue cycle management (RCM), 30
    revenue enhancement, 32
Financial Risks
    billing, coding, and collection problems, 254
    declining margins, 255
    ineffective patient retention, 255
    labor and supply cost increases, 254
    reimbursement changes, 254
FMLA. See Family Medical Leave Act
Functional Benchmarking. See Process Benchmarking
Future Trends, 44

G
Generation X (1965-1980), 110
Generation Z (1997-2012), 111
Generational Differences in Workforce, 110
Google Analytics, 212
Google My Business (GMB), 201

H
HAI. See Healthcare-Associated Infection
Health Apps, 237
    provider recommendations, 238
Health Information Exchange (HIE)
    benefits, 227
    challenges, 228
    data security and encryption, 229
    defined, 227
    patient consent and authorization, 229
Health Information Systems, 28
    continuous improvement, 29
    customize technology, 28
    electronic health record (EHR), 28
    Practice Management Systems (PMS), 28
Health Information Technology (Health IT), 221, 245
    mobile health apps, 245
    remote patient monitoring, 245
    telehealth, 245
    wearable devices, 245
Health Insurance Portability and Accountability Act (HIPAA), 35, 228
Healthcare Delivery Models
    concierge (private pay) medicine, 123
    fee-for-service, 121
    partnerships, 123
    population-based payments, 122
    value-based, 121
Healthcare-Associated Infection (HAI), 252
HIPAA. See Health Insurance Portability and Accountability Act
HIPAA for Professionals, 35
Human Hierarchy of Needs, 82

I
Incident Response
    documentation, 276
    investigation, 276
    non-punitive approach, 275
    protocols and procedures, 276
Independent Physicians, 84
Independent Practice Association (IPA), 89
    collective purchasing power, 90
    conflict of interest, 90
    contract negotiation, 90
    limited control, 90
    loss of autonomy, 90
    network access, 89
    pros and cons, 89
    regulatory compliance, 90

Index

Infection Control Measures, 273
Interoperability Strategies
  application programming interface (API), 226
  middleware software, 225
  open source benefits, 226
  standardized data exchange, 226
IPA. *See* Independent Practice Association
ISO 31000, 262

K
Key Performance Indicators (KPIs), 36, 129, 168, 211
Key Players to Achieve Success
  administrative staff, 8
  allied professionals, 7
  executive committees, 8
  governing boards, 8
  nurses, 7
  patients and families, 8
  physicians and clinicians, 7
  support staff, 8
Keys to Selecting Staffing-Models
  flexibility and adaptability, 49
  patient-centered staffing, 49
  skill mix, 50
  technology integration, 50
KPIs. *See* Key Performance Indicators

L
Labor Laws, 65
Lean and Six Sigma, 10
  Lean, 10
  Lean vs Six Sigma, 11
  manufacturing principles, 10
  Six Sigma, 11
Lean Six Sigma, 37
Legal Compliance, 35
  Affordable Care Act (ACA), 35
  Health Insurance Portability and Accountability Act (HIPAA), 35

Legal Risks
  alleged negligence or misdiagnosis, 255
  compliance failures, 255
  contract disputes, 255
  patient data protection, 255
Locum Tenens Work, 100

M
Managed Care Contracting, 125
Management Collaboratives, 181
Manufacturing Principles. *See* Lean and Six Sigma
Market Research Methods
  competitor analysis, 196
  digital analytics, 196
  focus groups, 196
  patient interviews, 196
  sample patient persona, 197
  surveys and questionnaires, 195
Marketing Analytics
  Google Analytics, 212
  identify trends, 212
  patient management systems, 212
  predictive analytics, 214
  ROI demonstration, 212
  social media analytics, 212
Marketing KPIs, 211
Mayo Clinic Values Council, 4
MCPI. *See* Lean and Six Sigma
Measure Efficiency and Performance, 36
  benchmarking, 36
  key performance indicators (KPIs), 36
Measures of Healthcare Quality
  access, 171
  patient-healthcare team relationships, 171
  technical quality, 172
Medical Consumer Price Index (MCPI), 143
Medication Management, 272
Merit-based Incentive Payment System (MIPS), 15

MGMA DataDive Operations Metrics, 44
Middleware Software, 225
Millennials (1981-1996), 110
Minimum Wage, 66
MIPS. *See* Merit-based Incentive Payment System
Mission, Vision, and Values
    clarity of purpose, 4
    culture building, 4
    goal alignment, 4
Mission, Vision, and Values Implementation
    define values, 5
    ensure consistency, 5
    envision the future, 5
    reflect on core purpose, 5
MVV. *See* Mission, Vision, and Values

N
Natural Language Processing (NLP), 61
Negative Patient Reviews, 209
NLP. *See* Natural Language Processing

O
Occupational Safety and Health Act (OSHA), 69
Operational Excellence, 10
Operational Leadership, 1
    mission statement, 2
    values, 3
    vision statement, 2
Operational Risks
    cyberattack, 254
    staffing shortages, 253
    supply chain disruptions, 254
    workflow inefficiencies, 253
Operational Staffing Indicators, 43
    employee productivity metrics, 43
    provider productivity metrics, 43
    staff turnover rate, 43
    staff-to-patient ratio, 43
    time-to-fill vacancies, 43

Organizational Design and Structure
    billing, 25
    finance, 25
    front office, 25
    human resources, 25
    informational technology (IT), 25
    marketing and public relations (PR), 26
    operations and facilities, 26
    performance improvement, 25
    quality assurance (QA), 25
    risk management, 26
    six decision-making factors, 27
OSHA. *See* Occupational Safety and Health Act
Outsourcing, 57
    automation, 57
    data security, 61
    impact assessment, 59
    non-core functions identified, 58
    phased implementation, 62
    revenue cycle, 59
    scheduling cycle, 59
    service level agreements, 58
Overtime Pay, 66

P
Patient Concerns and Inquiries, 279
Patient Engagement, 33
Patient Identification Processes, 273
Patient Online Reviews, 209
Patient Pre-Visit Activities, 125
Patient Referral Programs
    enhance patient experience, 206
    program implementation, 207
    referral incentivizing, 207
    relationships with fellow professionals, 206
Patient Registration Activities, 126
Patient Safety Initiatives, 272
Patient Safety Practices
    data security, 271
    interoperability, 271

Index

resistance to change and reporting, 270
standardization and training, 271
Patient Satisfaction Surveys, 37
Payer Contracting Review
    contract performance, 136
    monthly, 138
    payer considerations, 146
    quarterly, 137
Payer KPIs, 137
Payer Negotiation Issues/Resolutions, 144
Payer Response to Proposal, 150
    break-even response, 151
    no response to request, 150
    proposal denial, 150
Payer Targets and Proposals, 141
Payment Management, 128
Pay-Per-Click (PPC), 204, 208
PHI. *See* Protected Health Information
Physician Burnout, 103
Physician Compensation, 113
Physician Employment Agreement Compensation Plan, 75
Physician Recruitment Expenses
    candidate travel fees, 106
    marketing fees, 106
    onboarding, 106
    relocation allowances, 106
    sign-on bonuses, 106
    tuition reimbursement, 106
Physician Retention, 100
Physician Shortages, 76, 101
Physician Turnover
    cost and disruption, 106
PMS. *See* Practice Management System
Post-Audit Improvement, 129
Posting a Staff Position, 51
Practice Management System (PMS), 32, 159, 162
Practice Profitability KPIs, 170
Predictive Analytics, 215
    AI-driven, 245

Predictive Analytics in Staffing. *See* Future Trends
Private Practice Ownership
    pros and cons, 88
Process Benchmarking
    benefits, 180
    functional benchmarking, 178
    management collaboratives, 181
    peer collaborations, 181
Process Improvement Tools, 12
    5 steps for clean, safe workspace, 12
    5 Whys, 12
    brainstorming, 12
    data analysis, 12
    identify, analyze, implement changes, 12
    spaghetti mapping, 12
    time observation, 12
    Value Stream Maps, 12
    waste walk and standard work, 12
    WEEDOUTS, 13
Protected Health Information (PHI), 228
Provider Engagement Surveys, 56

Q
Quality Assurance Audits, 269
Quality Improvement Strategy, 10

R
RCM. *See* Revenue Cycle Management
Recruitment Strategies
    applicant tracking system (ATS), 52
    behavioral or situational interviewing, 53
    branding, 51
    candidate-referral incentives, 53
    COVID-19 pandemic, 51
    online presence, 52
    patient testimonials, 52
    positive reputation, 51
    standardized interview questions, 52

talent acquisition channels, 52
team building, 52
video interviews, 52
Regulatory Compliance, 35
Regulatory Requirements
   CMS regulations, 274
   HIPAA compliance, 274
   OSHA standards, 274
   state and federal laws, 274
   VAERS reporting, 274
Remote Patient Monitoring (RPM), 229
Remote Therapeutic Monitoring (RTM), 229
Remote Work Model, 91
Retention, Burnout, and Turnover Metrics, 107
   diversity and inclusion, 108
   exit interviews, 109
   geographical distribution, 109
   mentorship programs, 108
   physician turnover rate, 108
   physician vacancy rate, 107
   physician-to-population ratio, 107
   satisfaction surveys, 108
   work-life balance, 109
Retention Strategies
   compensation strategy, 53
   employee dissatisfaction, 54
Return on Investment (ROI), 211-212
Revenue Cycle KPIs, 170
Revenue Cycle Management (RCM)
   chart documentation, 125
   claim production, 125
   contracting, 124
   denial management, 125
   post-audit improvement, 125
   pre-visit activities, 124
   receivables management, 125
   registration activities, 124
Revenue Cycle Team Meeting, 138
Risk Analysis
   Failure Mode and Effect Analysis (FMEA), 259
   Root Cause Analysis (RCA), 260
   SWOT Analysis, 259
Risk Awareness Training, 279
Risk Management
   documentation, 278
   limited resources, 272
   patient safety initiatives, 272
Risk Management Frameworks
   ISO 31000, 262
   traditional ERM frameworks, 261
   value-based ERM frameworks, 261
Risk Management Matrix, 258
Risk Management Plan Template
   communication and documentation, 267
   compliance, 267
   executive summary, 265
   improvement plans, 267
   incident response, 266
   management governance, 265
   mitigation strategies, 266
   monitor and evaluate, 267
   risk assessment, 266
   risk identification, 266
   templates and forms, 268
Risk Management Spectrum
   clinical risks, 252
   financial risks, 254
   legal risks, 255
   operational risks, 253
Risk Management Steps
   monitor and review, 257
   risk analysis, 256
   risk evaluation, 256
   risk identification, 256
   risk mitigation strategies, 257
ROI. *See* Return on Investment
Root Cause Analysis (RCA), 260
RPM. *See* Remote Patient Monitoring
RPM Technologies, 233
   early detection of health issues, 234
   personalized care plans, 235

Index

reduction in emergency room visits, 235
RTM. *See* Remote Therapeutic Monitoring

S
Search Engine Optimization (SEO), 193
Service Level Agreement (SLA), 58
SIPOC. *See* Suppliers, Inputs, Process, Outputs, Customers
SLA. *See* Service Level Agreement
SMART Marketing Goals
    specific, measurable, attainable, relevant, 211
Spaghetti Mapping, 12
Staff Turnover Causes, 113
Staffing Model Optimization, 45
    cost management, 45
    cultural fit, 46
    flexibility and adaptability, 46
    recruitment and retention, 45
    training, 46
Staffing Model Types, 46
    flexible staffing models, 47
    outsourcing options, 47
    team-based models, 47
    technology-enhanced models, 47
    traditional models, 46
Standardize Work Processes, 12
Suppliers, Inputs, Process, Outputs, Customers (SIPOC), 9
    tool to identify key stakeholders, 9
Surgical Safety Checklists, 272
SWOT Analysis
    opportunities and threats, 259
    strengths and weaknesses, 259

T
Telehealth Model, 92
    Consolidated Appropriations Act, 2023, 93
Telemedicine
    integration strategies, 231
    protocols, 232

provider resistance, 236
remote patient monitoring (RPM), 230
remote therapeutic monitoring (RTM), 230
technological barriers, 236
value demonstration, 237
Temporary Placeholder Work. *See* Locum Tenens Work
Title VII of Civil Rights Act
    2023 changes, 68

V
Vaccine Adverse Event Reporting System (VAERS), 274
VAERS. *See* Vaccine Adverse Event Reporting System
Value Proposition Components
    clarity, 199
    collaboration goals, 148
    market position, 147
    mission statement, 148
    questions and next steps, 148
    relevance, 199
    uniqueness, 199
Value Stream Maps, 12
Virginia Mason Institute
    Lean Pioneer, 14
    Waste Walk, 14
VSM. *See* Value Stream Maps

W
Website Building, 202
WEEDOUTS, 13
    defects or errors, 13
    excess motion, 13
    excess transportation, 13
    overproducing, 13
    staffing, 13
    too much material, 13
    unnecessary processing, 13
    waiting, 13
Work-Life Balance, 56

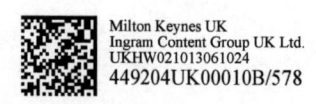

Milton Keynes UK
Ingram Content Group UK Ltd.
UKHW021013061024
449204UK00010B/578